Governing Public Hospitals

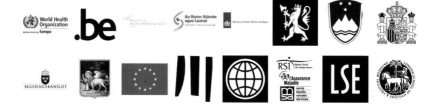

The European Observatory on Health Systems and Policies supports and promotes evidence-based health policy-making through comprehensive and rigorous analysis of health systems in Europe. It brings together a wide range of policy-makers, academics and practitioners to analyse trends in health reform, drawing on experience from across Europe to illuminate policy issues.

The European Observatory on Health Systems and Policies is a partnership between the World Health Organization Regional Office for Europe, the Governments of Belgium, Finland, Ireland, the Netherlands, Norway, Slovenia, Spain, Sweden and the Veneto Region of Italy, the European Commission, the European Investment Bank, the World Bank, UNCAM (French National Union of Health Insurance Funds), the London School of Economics and Political Science, and the London School of Hygiene & Tropical Medicine.

Governing Public Hospitals

Reform strategies and the movement towards institutional autonomy

Edited by

Richard B. Saltman, Antonio Durán, Hans F.W. Dubois

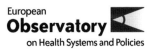

European
Observatory
on Health Systems and Policies

Keywords:
HOSPITALS, PUBLIC – trends
HOSPITAL ADMINISTRATION
HEALTH CARE REFORM
STRATEGIC PLANNING
EUROPE

Address requests about publications to: Publications, WHO Regional Office for Europe, Scherfigsvej 8, DK-2100 Copenhagen Ø, Denmark.

Alternatively, complete an online request form for documentation, health information, or for permission to quote or translate, on the Regional Office web site (http://www.euro.who.int/pubrequest).

ISBN 978 92 890 0254 7

Printed in the United Kingdom

Cover design by M2M

Contents

Preface

For hospital governance to be effective, it must incorporate two powerful and well-developed lines of health sector logic: on the one hand, national health policy and objectives; on the other, operational hospital management. One sphere is political, the other is technical. One is subjective and value based, the other is objective, with performance that can be measured both clinically and financially. The challenge for hospital-level governance is to integrate these two disparate logics into a coherent and effective institutional-level strategy.

This study explores key developments in public hospital governance in Europe. In doing so, it highlights the central role of hospital-level decision-making and how it is shaped by the various participants and stakeholders. In particular, it examines the degree to which granting an individual hospital the ability to make its own strategic, financial and clinical decisions – to become semi-autonomous within the public sector – may improve institutional-level functioning and outcomes.

In the initial chapters of this study, we draw on a substantial body of literature in a number of related health policy, public management and institutional governance arenas. How these different concepts might apply to public hospitals is the subject of considerable discussion here. It is in the interface of these differing conceptual approaches, with the evidence and experience seen in the eight country cases, that we catch a glimpse of the future of public hospital governance in Europe. We hope that this study can serve as a solid conceptual and practical contribution to future quantitative as well as qualitative research on this important subject.

Richard B. Saltman, Antonio Durán
and Hans F.W. Dubois

Acknowledgements

The editors are grateful to the substantial number of individuals and institutions that helped to produce this volume in a relatively short period of time.

First, we thank our country case study authors, who worked under tight deadlines and produced the empirical information upon which this volume is based. We also want to express our gratitude to Arturo Álvarez, who contributed substantially to the ideas on governance developed in Chapters 1 and 2. Additionally, we are grateful to the Andalusian School of Public Health in Granada, which hosted the author's workshop, as well as to the Regional Government of Andalusia, which provided support for that meeting. Further, we would like to thank Josep Figueras of the European Observatory on Health Systems and Policies, Pascal Garel of the Hope Foundation and Hans Maarse (also one of our case study authors), all of whom read the first draft of Part I and participated in a Brussels-based meeting that provided important comments and suggestions. A subsequent draft was further reviewed by Nigel Edwards, Hans Maarse and Pascal Garel. We also benefited greatly from testing Chapter 3 at a meeting of the European Health Policy Group in Paris, hosted by IRDES, and at which the comments by the discussant Nick Mays and by the participants helped us to shape our conceptual and practical approach. An early seminar at the London School of Economics and Political Science (LSE) was essential in helping to develop our thinking, and Champa Heidbrink and LSE also graciously provided rooms for a series of editors' meetings as the study took shape.

While none of the above-mentioned parties are in any way responsible for how we used their wisdom and support, we are very grateful to them for their assistance in making this what we hope will be a useful contribution to the growing literature on hospital governance.

Richard B. Saltman, Antonio Durán
and Hans F.W. Dubois

List of tables, figures and boxes

Tables

Figures

Boxes

List of abbreviations

AB	(Hospital) Administration Board
AC	Autonomous Community (Spain)
APSH	Administrative Public Sector Hospitals
BMS	Medical Staff Board (Netherlands)
CAHS	Central Health System Administration
CEO	chief executive officer
CIPFA	Chartered Institute of Public Finance and Accountancy
CZK	Czech koruna
DGTF	Directorate-General of Treasury and Finance (Portugal)
DRG	diagnosis-related group
DTC	diagnosis–treatment combination
EHIF	Estonian Health Insurance Fund
EU	European Union
GP	general practitioner
HMP	Hospital Master Plan
IT	information technology
ITC	independent treatment centre
IVF	in vitro fertilization
JWO	Jewish Women's Organization
MRI	magnetic resonance imaging
NHS	National Health Service
NKr	Norwegian krone
NPM	new public management
OAPMH	Official Accounting Plan of the Ministry of Health

OECD	Organisation for Economic Co-operation and Development
PEEH	Public enterprise entity hospitals
PFI	Private Finance Initiative
PPPH	Public–private partnership hospital
PCT	Primary Care Trusts
RHA	Regional Health Administration (Portugal)
SHA	Strategic health authority
SHI	Social health insurance
SNS	Spanish National Health System
UCLH	University College London Hospitals

List of contributors

Authors

Arturo A. Álvarez is Senior Consultant at Técnicas de Salud in Seville.

David Chinitz is Associate Professor of Health Policy and Management at the School of Public Health of the Hebrew University of Jerusalem.

Hans F.W. Dubois was Assistant Professor at Kozminski University in Warsaw at the time of writing, and is now Research Officer at Eurofound in Dublin.

Antonio Durán is Chief Executive Officer of Técnicas de Salud in Seville.

Nigel Edwards was Director of Policy & Communications and Acting Chief Executive Officer at the NHS Confederation in London at the time of writing, and is now Senior Fellow, Kings Fund and Director of Global Health Reform at KPMG LLP.

Jarno Habicht is Head of the WHO Country Office in the Republic of Moldova and former Head of the WHO Country Office in Estonia.

Triin Habicht is Head of the Health Care Department of the Estonian Health Insurance Fund in Tallinn.

Ana P. de Jesus Harfouche is Hospital Manager at the Portuguese Oncology Institute "Francisco Gentil" in Lisbon.

Pavel Hroboň is Fellow at the Advance Healthcare Management Institute in Prague.

Maris Jesse is Director of the Estonian National Institute for Health Development in Tallinn.

Léon Lodewick is former interim Chief Executive Officer in several Dutch hospitals, adviser of government and of Supervisory Boards in the Netherlands.

Hans Maarse is Professor of Health Policy and Administration of the Faculty of Health, Medicine and Life Sciences of the University of Maastricht.

Jon Magnussen is Professor of Health Services Research/Health Economics at the Department of Public Health and General Practice of Norwegian University of Science and Technology in Trondheim.

Vítor M. dos Reis Raposo is Assistant Professor at the Faculty of Economics of the University of Coimbra.

Tomas Roubal is Health Policy Analyst at the Czech Republic Ministry of Health in Prague.

Richard B. Saltman is Associate Head of Research Policy at the European Observatory on Health Systems and Policies, and Professor of Health Policy and Management at the Rollins School of Public Health of Emory University in Atlanta.

Introduction: innovative governance strategies in European public hospitals

Richard B. Saltman, Antonio Durán and Hans F.W. Dubois

This book explores innovative strategies in how acute-care public hospitals are managed in eight differently structured health systems – seven European systems and Israel. While these strategies reflect different national circumstances and needs, there appear to be three connected factors driving this organizational realignment: first, rapid technological improvement in clinical and informational capacity among hospitals generally (both public and private); second, growing patient expectations regarding quality, safety, responsiveness and choice concerning health care providers; and consequently, third, growing political pressures on public authorities to restructure the command and control relationships embedded within traditional governance models of publicly owned institutions. While the first development has generated new managerial needs and possibilities within public hospitals, the second has served to push national health policy-makers to consider new organizational approaches to ensure that publicly owned hospitals provide the range and standard of clinical services that the citizenry increasingly expect, as countries become wealthier and societies become more middle class (Saltman & von Otter, 1992).

Through the late 1980s, publicly owned hospitals in Europe were predominantly focused on delivering acute medical care, including emergency and scheduled elective inpatient procedures, and also (in many countries) on treating a wide range of less serious acute conditions in outpatient clinics (Healy & McKee, 2002). During this period, efforts to coordinate care at various service delivery levels were not well articulated, especially between intra-mural and extra-mural care. The central emphasis for public hospitals was placed on the importance of equity of access to appropriate clinical care for all residents/ citizens, regardless of income or profession. Additionally, these institutions were viewed (in tax-funded Beveridge health systems) as a central element within a larger system of public responsibility for public health, and were linked to other public services at the local level, which were expected jointly to provide the necessary individual services (especially to children and elderly) as well as collective preventive services (Healy & McKee, 2002). In the view of many commentators, these equity-oriented efforts were highly successful from a population-based epidemiological perspective, certainly compared with the less systematic, less population-based services of the earlier post-Second World War period (Holland, Olsen & Florey, 2007).

Although the 1978 Alma Ata Declaration had emphasized the importance of primary health care in health systems development, efforts to prioritize the role of primary care services and primary health care services in developed countries were only in their initial stages (Saltman, Rico & Boerma, 2006). Similarly, discussions regarding how better to integrate chronic and elderly care services across primary care and hospital sectoral boundaries also were still at the point of exploring alternative organizational solutions (Nolte & McKee, 2008).

Major organizational change in how public hospitals were governed began in the late 1980s (Sweden) and the early 1990s (England), with a wave of health system reforms triggered by efficiency and quality concerns (Saltman & Figueras, 1997). Drawing on new management strategies taken from private industry, these reforms sought to introduce more flexible service delivery arrangements, seeking governance models that could stimulate greater institutional autonomy and, in turn, more effective integration across different types of services. In its initial stages, this reform process was highly contested, particularly by defenders of the traditional public system, who viewed the changes as politically driven (Dahlgren, 1994; Pollock, 2004). Over the ensuing years, however, many of these reforms have been "normalized" and have increasingly been seen as simply one potentially useful element within a broader spectrum of hospital management approaches (Saltman, 2009).

During this same period, the applied field of "governance" theory emerged in the academic world. A number of different social science disciplines (e.g. sociology, economics, political science, public administration, management, organizational theory) have each sought to articulate their own particular theoretical perspective on the process of governance in the public sector. These widely varying academic efforts have now transformed what had been an undifferentiated if somewhat vague notion into an umbrella concept that incorporates a broad range of public sector decision-making activities. Reflecting this development, there is now a substantial body of social policy literature around a general notion of sectoral and institutional governance which reflects numerous social phenomena and thus has the potential to support multiple policy solutions for public sector institutions.

One useful overview of this broader understanding of public sector governance strategies can be seen in Table 0.1. This framework contrasts structural characteristics of the traditional Weberian (post-Second World War) bureaucratic state – in many respects the baseline notion of formal governance in Europe – with the considerably more diffuse approach to governance that subsequently has emerged in the new (post-cold war) "postmodern" state.

Table 0.1 *Characteristics of bureaucratic versus postmodern states*

Weberian bureaucratic state	A postmodern state
Government	Governance
Hierarchy (Weberian)	Heterarchy (networks etc.)
Power (1): zero-sum game	Power (1): positive-sum game
Power (2): concentrated	Power (2): diffuse
Elitist	Pluralist
Unitary, centralized, monolithic state	Decentralized, fragmented, hollowed-out state
Strong, central executive	Segmented executive
Clear lines of accountability	Blurred lines of accountability
State central control	State central steering
Single homogeneous public service ethos	Heterogeneous service cultures

Source: Richards & Smith, 2002.

This broader "postmodern" approach to state governance has direct implications for how policy and decision-making activities are conceived and conducted within publicly operated health systems across Europe. Over the initial decade of health sector reforms during the 1990s, research studies tended to focus on the ability of specific health sector reforms to improve overall performance in terms of key objectives, such as equity, efficiency and competition (Glennerster, Owens & Matsaganis, 1994; Jönsson, 1994; Robinson & Le Grand, 1994; Harrison & Calltorp, 2000). The ability to improve outcomes on these objectives has been applied particularly to assess changes in decision-making strategies within the hospital sector. More recently, however, health policy researchers have begun to turn away from content-focused evaluation to consider the impact of the underlying process-oriented frameworks that steer and constrain overall health reform behaviour (WHO, 2000; Mossialos et al., 2010). Underlying both successful and not-so-successful reform strategies are substantially different approaches to what has now been termed *hospital governance* in Europe.

The term "hospital governance" is somewhat complicated to apply. Policy-makers as well as economists traditionally have tended to view key elements of hospital performance through the related but narrower lens of "hospital management". Moreover, the term governance, like other, similar English-language terms relating to directing policy (e.g. stewardship and accountability), does not easily translate into some European languages, so that the concept of governance itself may have different meanings in different national contexts. Both conceptually and practically, then, the term "hospital governance" may have structural limitations as a description of new concepts and institutional arrangements for public hospitals.

As currently used, the process-focused notion of "hospital governance" encompasses three different levels of hospital-related decision-making. Each level has its own distinct characteristics, with its own separate group of decision-makers. All three levels interact with each other in complex patterns that then define the actual "governance structure" for hospitals, and in particular for the publicly owned hospitals that are the subject of this study.

At what can be termed the "macro" level, there are national government decisions that determine the basic structure, organization and finance of the entire health care system, and of the hospital sector within it. The decision to maintain publicly operated, tax-funded hospitals, for example, is just such a "macro governance" decision. The parameters of this macro level differ notably in different country contexts, with the range and specificity of requirements and regulations that fall under "macro governance" varying considerably between countries. Moreover, in some countries, for some types of policy decisions, authority may be devolved to regional or even local governments. What is seen as appropriate regulatory rule-making for public hospitals in one country (for instance, England) may not be seen as appropriate state behaviour within another system (such as Spain). Moreover, from a centralizing viewpoint, an increasing proportion of these macro decisions are now being made by European Union level institutions (Mossialos et al., 2010). Taken overall, then, the macro level of hospital governance is the part of traditional national, regional and/or supranational policy-making that establishes the structural, organizational and operational architecture of the hospital sector.

An intermediate "meso" level of hospital governance is focused on decision-making at the overall institutional level of the hospital. In some instances (see the Norwegian case study in Chapter 10), this level may incorporate two or more physically separate hospital sites that operate as a single corporate entity. The meso level focuses on the senior decision-makers for each separately operated hospital. As the eight case studies in this volume demonstrate, in a growing number of countries, decision-making at this meso level for public hospitals has been lodged in a separate institutional supervisory board and with the hospital's chief executive officer (CEO). To a degree, these publicly operated hospitals increasingly have a meso-level governance structure that resembles that of a private company. It is at this meso level that all important organizational policy decisions that the hospital is allowed to make (e.g. that are not restricted by macro-level regulatory constraints) are made.

Lastly, the "micro" level of hospital governance focuses on the day-to-day operational management of staff and services inside the organization. This level of "governance" is in fact what has traditionally been known as "hospital management" and incorporates such subsets as personnel management, clinical quality assurance, clinic-level financial management, patient services and hotel services (cleaning services, catering, etc.).

This broad conceptual framework of macro, meso and micro levels of hospital governance serves a variety of useful purposes. First, it clarifies and specifies the large number of different activities that contribute to the governance process in the hospital sector. Second, for publicly operated hospitals in particular, it separates out the three levels of decision-making that often get commingled and/or confused within traditional state-run health systems.

Third, regarding this volume, the framework clearly categorizes the aspects of hospital governance that are the subject of consideration here. Since all three levels – macro, meso and micro – interact with each other and contribute to overall hospital governance, they all receive some degree of attention in the chapters of Part I that follow. However, this book does not focus on or emphasize either the macro, state policy-making dimension or the micro, intra-organizational managerial dimension of hospital governance. Rather, the main purpose of this volume is to better understand the meso-level, whole hospital aspect of governance and how it has changed in a set of countries with predominantly publicly operated hospitals over the past two decades of health sector reform in Europe.

This decision to concentrate on the meso level reflects several factors. There is already a large body of literature available about both the macro level e.g. state health system decision-making, and the micro level e.g. technical intra-hospital management. While both of these dimensions are clearly essential to building a full picture of hospital governance, they reflect areas of decision-making for which considerable analysis has already been conducted and can be drawn upon. Moreover, given the high degree of interrelationship among these three dimensions, a better understanding of meso-level hospital decision-making is essential to a proper picture of the entire governance process.

Further, it is at the meso level of hospital governance that some of the more interesting and innovative reforms have been carried out in publicly operated hospitals across Europe. Seven of the eight case studies in Part II, which serve as the basis for analysis in Part I, are taken from countries that have been at the forefront of efforts to redesign meso-level hospital governance. The eighth, Netherlands, has a meso-level governance structure composed entirely of non-profit-making private hospitals and thus can serve as an outer benchmark for how far the process of meso-level change has proceeded within the other seven publicly operated hospital systems.

This meso-level process of change in hospital governance has to date received insufficient analytical attention. As Chapters 3 and 4 highlight, there is a considerable amount to be learned regarding what has changed at the institutional level of hospital governance, and the extent to which the changes have achieved their intended objectives.

Lastly, and self-evidently for many European readers, the preponderance of hospital systems in many parts of Europe (northern, southern and central) are some form of publicly owned and operated institutions.

The interest among national policy-makers in reforms introduced at this meso level continues to be strong in a number of European countries. Countries that have introduced meso-level structural reforms of their public hospitals are interested in learning what other countries have done, and how well it has worked. Other countries that are currently contemplating meso-level reform are interested in knowing more about the strategies, mechanisms and results from existing reform efforts.

Within this meso level of hospital governance, this study has restricted its focus on several important parameters. As already noted, the study concentrates almost entirely (with the exception of the Netherlands) on countries in which all or nearly all hospitals are publicly owned and operated. In addition, these hospitals are publicly funded, either via tax revenues or (in Estonia and the Czech Republic) through social insurance funds, which in the hybrid central European model, are administered or closely controlled by national government agencies. Other than the Netherlands, this volume does not consider or evaluate meso-level hospital governance in traditional social insurance countries in western Europe. Furthermore, given its focus on changes within publicly operated hospitals, this study does not discuss or assess hospital governance issues with regard to private profit-making hospitals neither in the eight case study countries, or elsewhere.[1]

As also noted earlier, the eight countries selected for the case studies have each implemented innovative reforms at the meso level of hospital governance. These reforms make their hospital governance experiences useful to compare, and valuable for national policy-makers and academics seeking to learn more about potential new meso-level strategies of hospital governance.

A further, methodological point is that this study is qualitative rather than quantitative in nature. The volume seeks to understand changes in the process of institutional-level decision-making for publicly operated hospitals, and the degree to which such changes are effective and/or sustainable over time. It does not incorporate quantitative efforts to evaluate micro-level management, nor does it attempt to assemble or review performance management data regarding hospital quality or clinical outcomes. While such quantitative, micro-level assessment is valuable for decision-making, its structure and mechanisms involve a different set of research methodologies from those utilized here (Smith et al., 2009).

Lastly, and importantly, this study focuses particular interest and attention on one central, controversial dimension of meso-level institutional governance – that is, the numerous recent reforms that seek to make public hospitals semi-autonomous, with their own separate Supervisory Boards and with considerable independence of decision-making. This pursuit of a viable model of semi-autonomous management inside the public hospital sector has been under way now since the late 1980s. Efforts to create self-sustaining models of "public firms" (Saltman & von Otter, 1992) or "quasi-markets" (Le Grand & Bartlett, 1993) in the public hospital sector began in the late 1980s in Sweden, and in April 1991 in England with the first wave of self-governing trusts. Magnussen rightly points out in his conclusions to the Norway case study (see Chapter 10) that the reality of macro-level hospital governance at the state level means that meso-level governance for public hospitals can never be more than "semi-autonomous". However, as Bevan has commented,[2] both the degree of decision-making autonomy enjoyed by these different meso-level models, as well as the tipping point at which governments begin to regret such grants and reassert their central authority (Saltman, 2008), inevitably differ based on national political conditions and the prevailing cultural expectations within each country.[3] Stated another way, variations in these semi-autonomous models across countries may well reflect differing degrees of "publicness" in

1 See Jeurissen (2010) for a recent overview of profit-making hospitals..

2 At a European Health Policy Group Meeting in Paris, 29 April 2010.

3 See the introduction to Saltman & Bergman (2005), along with Vrangbaek (2007).

their mandates, and in the public/private mix of mechanisms, obligations, restrictions and incentives involved (Saltman, 2003).

This question of institutional autonomy within the public hospital sector may have implications that go beyond service structure and perceived financial effectiveness. Several recent academic analyses have suggested that autonomous institutional decision-making is associated with higher quality micro-level clinical outcomes (Bloom et al., 2010). While this finding is of great interest to policy-makers, this volume, as noted earlier, focuses on qualitative issues at the meso level rather than quantitative issues at the micro level.

One additional element of hospital semi-autonomy as used in this study is that it refers to a recognized, legitimate institutional status. In all eight country cases presented in Part II, publicly owned hospitals have acquired this semi-autonomous status as part of a formal governmental decision, typically national, but in some cases (e.g. Spain) regional in character. In the one country (Israel) where public hospitals have only a de facto rather than an institutional form of autonomy, the portion of their activities that is semi-autonomous is governed by a national government agreement to allow their outpatient clinics to operate as "Health Corporations". Thus, in all eight instances, semi-autonomy is a government-granted, more-or-less official status.

In turn, this separates the type of semi-autonomy discussed in this volume from measures taken by some hospital managements in some countries that, for whatever reason, are outside the normal decision-making channels. Such unsupervised activity can be for positive (as well as less positive) reasons; for example, crisis generated or to get around official rules that would prevent an effective response to an immediate need for services. Nonetheless, this is not an example of institutional semi-autonomy, but rather one of evading constricting regulations or procedures.[4]

This distinction between a formal institutional grant of autonomy and the de facto creation of a zone of independent action is important to an understanding of the evidence reported here. This study explores how public hospitals handle official authority granted to them by their owners to make institutional-level decisions, not the degree to which public hospitals evade formal controls that their managers find constraining and/or do not like.

Following from these observations, this study has two linked objectives. The first is to examine the core characteristics of governance theory generally, and to distill those elements that might be usefully applied to publicly operated hospitals. In keeping with this objective, Chapter 1 examines the changing

---

4   See Crozier (1971) for the classic discussion of how employees can manipulate rule-based management in public sector institutions.

position of the hospital in society, as well as the general concepts of governance theory, as developed by social scientists to address public policy issues generally. Chapter 2 then seeks to apply the key elements of this general theory of governance to the specific situation and conditions of governance within the hospital sector. It presents a four-part framework for analysing specifically meso-level hospital governance. Both of these chapters provide substantial references to existing literature, and in doing so seek to define the conceptual context within which national policy-makers in different countries develop their own strategy for reforming meso-level hospital governance.

The second objective of the book is to map innovative models of semi-autonomous public hospital governance adopted by European countries, and to explore the structure of these different models with regard to operating and decision-making autonomy. This objective is pursued through the eight national case studies presented in Part II. The different models that countries have established, the differing degrees to which these models reflect broader policy and management strategies in the health sector and, to a limited extent, the degree to which these differing models have achieved their intended organizational outcomes, are assessed in Chapters 3 and 4. Extensive comparative tables that document the degrees of similarity and dissimilarity in the case study responses to the questions asked by the editors can be found in the Appendix at the end of Chapter 4. The detail of these differing approaches is provided to enable both researchers and policy-makers to dig more deeply into the specifics of each semi-autonomous model.

These four initial chapters, dealing first with the theory and then subsequently with current strategies to reform hospital governance, form Part I of this volume. Those readers who would like more detailed information regarding current semi-autonomous models will find it in the eight country case studies presented in Part II.

References

Bloom N et al. (2010). *Why good practices really matter in healthcare*. London, VoxEU.org, Centre for Economic Policy and Research (http://www.voxeu.org/index.php?q=node/5939, accessed 2 May 2011).

Crozier M (1971). *The bureaucratic phenomenon*. Chicago, IL, University of Chicago Press.

Dahlgren G (1994). *Framtidens Sjukvardsmarknader – vinnare och förlorare? [Health care markets of the future – winners and losers?]*. Stockholm, Natur och Kultur.

Glennerster H, Owens P, Matsaganis M (1994). *Implementing GP fundholding.* Buckingham, Open University Press.

Harrison M, Calltorp J (2000). The re-orientation of market-oriented reforms in Swedish healthcare. *Health Policy*, 50:219–240.

Healy J, McKee M (2002). The role and functions of hospitals. In: McKee M, Healy J, eds. *Hospitals in a changing Europe.* Buckingham, Open University Press:59–80.

Holland WW, Olsen J, Florey C du V, eds. (2007). *The development of epidemiology.* Oxford, Oxford University Press.

Jeurissen P (2010). *For-profit hospitals* [doctoral thesis]. Rotterdam, Erasmus University Rotterdam Press.

Jönsson E (1994). *Har den sk Stockholmsmodellen genererat mer vård för pengarna? En jämförande utvärdering [Has the Stockholm model generated more care for the money? A comparative evaluation].* Stockholm, IKE.

Le Grand J, Bartlett W, eds. (1993). *Quasi-markets and social policy.* Basingstoke, MacMillan Press.

Mossialos E et al. (2010). *Health systems governance in Europe: the role of European Union law and policy.* Cambridge, Cambridge University Press.

Nolte E, McKee M (2008). *Caring for people with chronic conditions: a health system perspective.* Maidenhead, Open University Press.

Pollock A (2004). *NHS plc: the privatisation of our health care.* London, Verso.

Richards D, Smith MJ (2002). *Governance and public policy in the UK.* Oxford, Oxford University Press.

Robinson R, Le Grand J, eds. (1994). *Evaluating the NHS reforms.* London, The King's Fund Institute.

Saltman RB (2003). The melting public–private boundary in European health care systems. *European Journal of Public Health*, 13(1):24–29.

Saltman RB (2008). Decentralization, re-centralization and future European health policy. *European Journal of Public Health*, 18(2):104–106.

Saltman RB (2009). The rise of pragmatism in state/market debate. *Health Economics, Policy and Law*, 4:479–488.

Saltman RB, Bergman, SE (2005). Renovating the commons: Swedish health care reform in perspective. *Journal of Health Politics, Policy and Law*, 30(1–2):253–275.

Saltman RB, Figueras J (1997). *European health care reform: analysis of current strategies*. Copenhagen, WHO Regional Office for Europe.

Saltman RB, von Otter C (1992). *Planned markets and public competition: strategic reform in northern European health systems*. Buckingham, Open University Press.

Saltman RB, Rico A, Boerma W, eds. (2006). *Primary care in the driver's seat? Organizational reform in European primary care*. Maidenhead, Open University Press.

Smith PC et al., eds. (2009). *Performance measurement for health system improvement: experiences, challenges and prospects*. Cambridge, Cambridge University Press.

Vrangbaek K (2007). Towards a typology for decentralization in health care. In: Saltman RB, Bankauskaite V, Vrangbaek K, eds. *Decentralization in health care: strategies and outcomes*. Maidenhead, Open University Press:44–62.

WHO (2000). *World health report 2000: health systems – improving performance*. Geneva, World Health Organization.

PART I
Hospital governance in Europe

Chapter 1

The evolving role of hospitals and recent concepts of public sector governance

Antonio Durán, Hans F.W. Dubois and Richard B. Saltman

The current debate regarding public hospital governance reflects the convergence of two parallel logics relating to institutional development. One is the role of the public hospital in society – a role which has evolved with increasing speed over the past century, and which today presents a new range of challenges to address. The second developmental logic is the broad area of governance theory in general, which has experienced a "great leap forward" in the last two decades, stimulated by the fall of the Soviet Union and the consequent realization that the process of public sector political governance needs to incorporate financially and technically sophisticated – as well as authoritative – allocative characteristics.

This chapter explores each of these two logics separately, as background to considering in Chapter 2 how they are combined and applied in relation to the particular concept of "hospital governance".

1.1 The changing role of hospitals

1.1.1 From waiting for death to organ transplantation

Two centuries ago, hospitals were "overcrowded, chaotic … the last place any respectable person would want to find themselves" (Rosenberg, 1987, p. 4).

Their main purpose was to help people die in the presence of God – hence their frequent architectonic structure, with an altar at the end of patients' wards. Hospitals were not by chance staffed by nun nurses, literally "Sisters of Mercy", and doctors had a very limited technical arsenal. Surgeons were to a great extent the inheritors of barbers, who in their extra time practised tooth extractions and amputations…without anaesthesia. Inhaled anaesthesia was used in England for the first time in 1846, seven years before John Snow administered it to Queen Victoria during the birth of her eighth and ninth children (Caton, 2000). Hospitals had no antisepsis, laboratory, radiology or pharmacology departments.

Things moved faster from the 1930s onwards with the discovery of penicillin and the development of antibiotics, combined with an improvement in hygiene and the systematization of medical knowledge. Small *cottage hospitals* – staffed by an increasingly specialized workforce and concentrating diagnostic as well as therapeutic technologies in purpose-specific buildings – became part of their communities and, for the first time, became a source of civic pride. Concentrating resources and professionals in the same building was a good step, based on three factors: (1) economies of scale (the bigger the work volume, the better the use of resources and the lower the unit costs – once an operations theatre has been installed, running it for more hours would distribute its costs over more cases); (2) economies of reach/scope (using existing infrastructures would allow the achievement of higher quality results – a hospital with good emergency services and specialties such as cardiology, neurology, etc. can treat severe child pathologies immediately after delivery); and (3) facilitating professional training and the diffusion of better practices and technological knowledge (Durán, 2009).

Health system development after the Second World War gave hospitals financial and functional strength, and they soon became the place of reference for treatment of infection, recovery from a severe wound, or delivering a baby with less risk. The 1962 Hospital Plan for England and Wales, for example, consecrated the *district general hospital* as provider of specialized care to a population of between 100 000 and 150 000 people, in terms of both day care and inpatient care relating to internal medicine, surgery, paediatrics, and obstetrics and gynaecology (Maybin, 2007). As the role of the person responsible for coordinating the efforts of people working in these organizations grew in magnitude and prestige, university-level professional training in hospital administration became available and high-powered administrators became customary. In response, an early commentator wrote, "[m]embers of hospital boards have learned and are learning that it pays to let their full-time representative handle the management of their institution and doctors are being asked to go through channels when they have requests for equipment or suggestions for improved services" (Lentz, 1957, p. 459). However, since a wide range of organizational activities involved health professionals, their role in hospital life continued to be critical (Weiner, Shortell & Alexander, 1997).

Modern hospitals have become increasingly important institutions for their communities, even as they faced fundamental changes in their service delivery patterns (McKee & Healy, 2002; Lee, Chen & Weiner, 2004). The first kidney transplant, the launching of beta-blockers, laser treatment, the first coronary bypass and the first heart transplant widened the scope of these hospitals to encompass increasingly complicated operations. Starting from the four key specialties already mentioned (internal medicine, surgery, paediatrics, and obstetrics and gynaecology), the modern general hospital has on staff some 40 specializations, designed to serve a population upwards of 250 000–300 000 people, and has come to be viewed as the place where "practically any treatment" can be delivered.

Through to the late 1980s, in most European countries that relied upon predominantly publicly operated hospitals, patients were assigned to a specific institution based on a system of catchment areas, and were expected to be treated by a specific clinic, not by a specific doctor. As an example, reflecting this organization-centred operating focus, in one large public Finnish hospital in the late 1980s, patients in outpatient clinics were given an appointment to the clinic (not to a specific doctor). Moreover, that appointment was for a half-day period (morning or afternoon session) during which time they were expected to wait for whichever physician might appear. When questioned about this very bureaucratic appointment pattern, a senior ophthalmological surgeon famously responded that a public hospital is like the army, with patients being happy when a doctor comes to see them (Saltman, 1987). In this Finnish publicly operated hospital (and most others), doctors and nurses were public employees – often with civil servant status, including permanent posts, strong union representation, nationally negotiated pay schedules and the expectation of a "job for life".

With regard to financing, up to the late 1980s most publicly operated hospitals received the entirety of their funding from one or another public budget, on an annually appropriated basis, and were required to return any operating surplus at the end of the budget year. Capital investment decisions were made by senior political actors as part of a regional or national planning process, and were financed exclusively from public revenue. Approval for capital investment, particularly for buildings and major structural renovations, typically took many years. In Finland in the 1980s, the working assumption was that "it takes 10 years to build a hospital", reflecting the extensive political effort required to get onto the list of approved projects, followed by the wait for an allocation from a limited pool of funds (Saltman, 1988).

In practice, publicly owned hospitals in Europe in the 1980s were run as an administrative arm of a national, regional or local government. Many European health systems were set up and/or matured within bureaucratic structures – for example, the "Weberian" model of public administration that modern states had been developing for almost two centuries (Richards & Smith, 2002, p. 18). This model envisaged a clear-cut separation between political decision-makers (ministers) in charge of formulating policies and a civil service responsible for providing direct advice to ministers, but with little outside consultation. Strategic decision-making was in the hands of the senior political officials for the sector, typically the national ministry of health. The hospital director was often (depending on the country) a politically connected official, frequently with little or no private sector managerial experience, and either in position for life or (again, depending on the country) until a shift in the ruling political parties took place.

1.1.2 Contemporary pressures for further hospital change

This broad picture of the post-Second World War public hospital came under a variety of new epidemiological, technological and political pressures in the final years of the 20th century. Success in prolonging life expectancy for decades slowly but firmly multiplied the number of patients with long-term conditions. In England in 2001, for example, long-term conditions affected 35% of the population (17.5 million out of 50 million people) and generated 80% of primary care consultations, as well as 66% of emergency hospital admissions (Degeling & Erskine, 2009). Furthermore, it was recognized that as people lived longer, they often suffered from more than one disease and concentrated their ills at the end of their lives (subsequently termed the "compression of morbidity") (Fries, 1980). The impact of these demographic and epidemiological changes on patterns of clinical care has become increasingly clear. For many of the same reasons that produced the concentration of technologies under the same roof, services available to many people with long-term conditions are still characterized by a high dependency on acute care, a singularly clinical focus, a reactive character, a fragmented and sporadic nature, a lack of emphasis on personal experience and only a residual relationship to community services and secondary prevention (Wilson, Buck & Ham, 2005).

In contrast to this fixed structural pattern of care, technological, organizational, medical and pharmaceutical progress, better anaesthetic procedures, laparoscopic and other less-invasive surgical procedures all made possible major changes in how services can be delivered (McKee & Healy, 2002). These improvements allowed faster recovery of the patient so that an increasing number of elective surgery and other clinical procedures could be delivered in day-surgery centres. For example, most cataract operations in Organisation for Economic Co-operation and Development (OECD) countries and around 85% of elective surgery cases in the United Kingdom are now carried out without an overnight stay in the hospital (OECD, 2008). Major pharmaceutical and biochemical progress has also been made in treating other conditions, such as diabetes (e.g. insulin pump, glycaemia measurement) (Nolte, Bain & McKee, 2006), while certain cancers are easier to manage, often with less need for expensive hospital support services (Halpern & Yabroff, 2008). Many treatments previously requiring continuous care by specialized professionals (e.g. prostheses, transplants, dialysis) are no longer exclusively hospital procedures. For example, during 2006 and 2007, National Clinical Directors of the United Kingdom Department of Health reporting on emergency, mental health and maternity services concluded that most of these could be delivered in primary care centres, intermediate institutions (similar to "polyclinics") and even at home – especially if telemedicine support was provided (Imison, Naylor & Maybin, 2008).

As a consequence, from a service delivery perspective, many health problems can now be treated in more than one type of health care facility. Hospitals are no longer the exclusive location for delivering numerous forms of routine surgical and medical care, nor are they the discreet independent institutions they were in the post-Second World War period. Indeed, most European countries have been reducing the number of acute beds for decades – especially in western Europe (WHO Regional Office for Europe, 2010; Durán, Lara & Van Waveren, 2006; Hensher & Edwards, 1999; Saltman & Figueras, 1997) – and public hospitals face new conflicting pressures that influence activity at every level of the institution. Hospitals are expected to provide a wide range of services across sectoral boundaries – not least in the fields of chronic care, elderly care services and other forms of what is now termed "integrated care" services. New hospital-wide programmes have been introduced in areas such as quality assurance and patient safety.

Moreover, beyond epidemiological and technological change, new consumer-based pressures on hospitals have emerged. Measures of patient satisfaction and an explicit set of patient rights, for example – including patients' expectation to be consulted by their physician on the treatment they will receive – have now been adopted in many countries. Public patients in many countries also have choice of hospital (Winblad & Ringard, 2009; Or et al., 2010). Initiatives to acquire quantitative, standardized and comparative information on the performance of hospitals (capacity, efficiency, waiting times, patient safety and quality) are widespread (Maarse & Normand, 2009). In England, those tasks are undertaken not only by government agencies (currently the Care Quality Commission), but also by private organizations, such as Dr Foster, which publishes annual ratings relating to health care organizations' performance (Dixon et al., 2010).

These new pressures have not always been welcomed. Some hospital staff resent the shift from treating acute patients on an inpatient basis to having to coordinate their work with other levels of care. No hospital can be autonomous and self-sufficient any longer in all spheres. Contemporary requirements for conducting high-quality scientific research, for example, are greater than the scope of any single institution, with clinical trials often requiring collaboration between multiple national and international medical institutions (Shortell & Kaluzny, 2006).

1.1.3 The emergence of "new public management"

Current changes go beyond technical service delivery issues, as hospitals and health systems face a radically different set of expectations from both patients and their citizens. In response to demands for greater operating efficiency and improved responsiveness to patients, a range of reforms included under the umbrella term "new public management" (NPM), or "new public administration" (Greenwood, Pyper & Wilson, 2002) have sought to stimulate entrepreneurial hospital management by relying on quasi-market forces rather than planning, and by introducing strong performance measurement and monitoring mechanisms (Hood, 1991; Andresani & Ferlie, 2006). Responding to these new pressures, public hospital governance structures in some countries have been reconfigured, by creating quasi-independent Supervisory Boards that could make a range of operating and financial decisions without obtaining direct political approval (Osborne & Gaebler, 1992; Kettl, 1993). Public hospital managers were hired, with professional skills as managers that politicians, civil servants and public administrators often lacked.

These NPM arrangements reflected not only changing clinical capabilities and expectations but also a fundamentally changed fiscal picture in the health sector, produced by the impact of the electronic revolution and economic globalization on the finances of European industrial companies (and, via revenue from taxes, on the financial capacity of the national, regional or local government owners of public hospitals). Put frankly, national policy-makers increasingly realized that publicly operated health care systems could only afford to maintain solidarity by dramatically ramping up the efficiency with which public institutions operate. Operating efficiency took on increasing urgency after the extended recession in the early 1990s. The two sharp recessions in the 2000s, coupled with a dramatically altered international trading and manufacturing environment due to the growing influence of China, India, Brazil, the Russian Federation and other smaller emerging economies, as well as political changes in central and eastern Europe related to the end of the communist era and the expansion of the EU, all served to reinforce the basic message. As a consequence, although publicly owned hospitals still received most or all of their funding from public revenue, national policy-makers have increasingly sought to introduce some form of purchaser–provider split, institutionally separating the public funder from public providers, providing funds according to a case-based formula (typically adjusted diagnosis-related groups (DRGs)) and, increasingly, tying those payments to activity and/or performance levels.

1.1.4 Implications for future hospital governance

In key technical, financial and political respects, the world of public hospitals in the second decade of the 21st century is fundamentally different from how it had been previously (Rechel et al., 2009). This perception, in turn, has led to a growing concern that the current historically inherited hospital model – in both structural and administrative terms – may not be sustainable over the coming decades (The Joint Commission, 2008). Hints about the hospital of the future indicate that some institutions will be smaller than the present ones but are more likely to concentrate on high-cost, lower frequency specialized and emergency care, and to focus more on efficiency, patient orientation and innovation than current specialized hospitals. In contrast, a second group of hospitals will concentrate on high-volume, single-specialty elective (routine) care. The first group – the smaller, multi-specialty hospitals – are expected to have rather unclear institutional borders compared with current hospitals, with a core of clinical facilities serving the most acute cases. They will be equipped with more operating theatres and emergency units and linked as a network by means of information technologies (IT). Moreover, the whole ensemble would be surrounded by services that are outsourced to a massive extent, including early discharge, "medi-hotels", home care, pathology, laboratory services, catering, laundry services, archives and so on (Braithwaite et al., 1995). While some health care facilities are already being built and operated partly with such an orientation (van Laarhoven, 2008), other voices warn against the risk of cost increases and poor quality stemming from loss of economies of scale (Sibbald, McDonald & Roland, 2007).

However the public hospital's structure and function evolves, a clear and transparent effort will be necessary in order to ensure quality and efficiency in the increasingly complex interventions kept inside the hospital walls, as well as in services decentralized from hospitals to the community and/or other organizations. Most of all, the situation will require better coordination between levels of care, better information tools and better strategies to ensure accountability by the multiple actors involved (Smith et al., 2009).

Such changing modalities of acute and elective clinical care, growing demands for integrated chronic and elderly care in the context of increased demand for patient voice and choice, and broader social changes, in turn, call for an overhaul of the way hospitals are led. In essence, hospitals will need to be governed as they in fact now operate – as part of a continuum or network of outpatient and inpatient care providers that are concerned with patient responsiveness and better attention to the role of professionals (Hoek, 2007). Increasingly, publicly operated hospitals will have to pursue their medical and social objectives (from improved performance to income and sustainability goals, knowledge development and prestige and social cohesion) by adapting the way they are governed to what will be new, post-NPM circumstances. Whatever else this transition may imply, one very clear conclusion is that the traditional, monolithic, command-and-control model of public hospital leadership will no longer be a viable approach to future hospital governance.

1.2 A brief review of governance theory

Having explored the changing organizational context and structure of public hospitals, this second part of the chapter reviews the development in public policy of a general theory of governance. While these two areas have different sources, together they serve as the reference base from which, in Chapter 2, we will examine the characteristics of specifically hospital-focused governance.

1.2.1 The concept of governance

A defining feature of the current era in western countries is the large number of actors and institutions involved in every publicly accountable policy process. In the past, "governing was basically regarded as one-way traffic from those governing to those governed" (Kooiman, 2000, p. 142). As the number of actors in the policy arena has multiplied, however, the boundaries between the public and private sectors have become more blurred and central government command over a much more complex policy process has receded (Peters, 2004). The key tenet is that "political power" no longer exclusively rests with formal political structures (Pierre, 2000). As one political scientist described the new environment, "The policy process is now crowded with more actors ... the government is hardly anymore the most powerful actor in the policy arena" (Alvarez-Rosete, 2007, p. 41). Instead of a top-down process of imposed political authority, the current policy process involves a large number of different actors.

Along lines similar to those in the basic framework presented in Table 0.1 in the Introduction, Newman (2001) suggests the following shifts in the dominant governance typology inside the public sector:

1. a move away from hierarchy and competition as alternative models for delivering services, towards networks and partnerships traversing the public, private and voluntary sectors;

2. recognizing the blurring of boundaries and responsibilities for tackling social and economic issues;

3. recognizing and incorporating policy networks into the process of governing;

4. replacing traditional models of command and control with "governing at a distance";

5. developing more reflexive and responsive policy tools;

6. a shifting of the role of government to a focus on providing leadership, building partnerships, steering and coordinating, and providing system-wide integration and regulation;

7. the emergence of "negotiated self-governance" within communities, cities and regions, based on new practices of coordinating activities through networks and partnerships;

8. opening up decision-making to greater participation by the public;

9. innovation in democratic practice as a response to problems relating to the complexity and fragmentation of authority, and the challenges this presents to traditional democratic models; and

10. a broadening of focus by government that goes beyond institutional concerns to encompass the involvement of civil society in the process of governance.

Several useful concepts derived from the general theory of governance can be identified in recent political science literature. Network governance (Kjær, 2004) is a concept that captures relationships between government and the governed, driven by specific needs or outcomes of "networked bargaining" in the context of reduced governmental authority. A policy network typically incorporates the interaction of both state and non-state organizations and individuals – from governmental departments and non-departmental public bodies to private companies, professional bodies, service providers, users of public services and so on – while seeking to shape agendas and decision-making, and remaining dependent upon each other for resources. Networks vary according to the subsector, the stage of the policy process, the issue at stake, the equilibrium of power, and so on. The policy network approach depicts a policy-making process that is far more complex and messy than those perceived by previous paradigms. Rhodes defined governance as the product of self-organized and interorganized networks (Rhodes, 1997a). In that context, government is only one subtype of a specific governance mechanism – the other types being markets, corporate hierarchies, clans, networks and formal law (Ezzamel & Reed, 2008). Usually, combinations of such mechanisms are understood to be required for effective governance (Rodríguez et al., 2007).

Governance comprises both formal structures – statutes, judicial decrees, administrative guidelines – and the informal exercise of judgement by the numerous actors involved in implementation. Any subset of rules, laws or practices reflects only part of a broader governance framework (Lynn, Heinrich & Hill, 2000). A comparative case study between the United Kingdom and Germany, for example (Kuhlmann, Allsop & Saks, 2009), shows that not only government and service users but also a variety of professional groups shape the nature and form of public control.

The tools and strategies used by stakeholders to achieve their policy objectives have also evolved and it is now commonplace to refer to governance as a range of old and new tools and instruments through which public policy goals may be achieved and/or delivered (Zito, Radaelli & Jordan, 2003; Hood, 2006). The very concept implies that the ways to govern the public sector and the tools for doing so have changed (Salamon, 2002) and – implicitly or explicitly – should change further from old command-and-control, public administration or management models (Bovaird & Löffler, 2003). This particular governance paradigm reflects the melting of distinctions between the political, managerial and administrative realms and between policy formulation and implementation in a crowded policy process with boundaries that are often blurred. Drawing on the conceptual language used in the Introduction, this new governance paradigm means that the macro, meso and micro dimensions of specifically public hospital governance interact within and between each other in complex ways that create patterns and networks of actors, rather than according to the old model of explicit hierarchical relationships of decision-makers and decision-takers.

1.2.2 A definition of governance

The term "governance" has a broad range of meanings (Rhodes, 1996; Stoker, 1997; van Doeveren, 2009). Rhodes argues that governance can take seven different forms, while Stoker claims that there are five, which emphasizes both the multi-dimensionality of the concept and some obvious lack of consensus. Meanings vary also across countries, languages, fields of research and specific authors. In the United States and Australia, governance retains its original meaning, referring to steering rather than *rowing* (Osborne & Gaebler, 1992), with Rhodes (1997b) even suggesting *steering* to be a synonym of *governance*. From a European perspective, however, the term is more identified as being aligned with "governing".

The definition proposed by the World Bank centres more narrowly on the issue of power and is universally applicable, defining governance as: "exercise of political power to manage a nation's affairs" (World Bank, 1989, p. 60). Addressing the relationship between governance and the economy, governance is seen as expressing "the steering capacities of a political system, the ways in which governing is carried out, without making any assumption as to which institutions or agents do the steering" (Gamble, 2000, p. 110). In Part One of their book *Governance, politics and the state*, Pierre & Peters (2000) suggest that the concept refers to:

- first, a *structure* (a mixed system of hierarchies, markets, networks and communities involved in the delivery of services);

- second, a *dynamic outcome* – that is, the processes of steering, coordinating and goal-setting through which society can only be governed nowadays; and

- third, a *theory* to help the policy analyst understand new developments in state–society relationships.

Much as the above range of definitions suggest about "governance" generally, the term *hospital governance* has been applied to a wide range of strategic and operational decision-making activities. This topic is developed further in Chapter 2 which focuses specifically on hospital governance.

1.2.3 Comparing governance and management

In addition to political science, the discipline of management also has placed considerable emphasis on defining governance. For almost three decades, the generic concept of management was challenged as being unable to capture what actually takes place in many organizations. High-profile commentators such as Jeffrey Pfeffer and Henry Mintzberg (Pfeffer, 1981; Mintzberg, 1983) contended that the key factors that influenced organizational decision-making were *leadership*, *power* and *politics*.

Organizations, they suggested, are more than just systems for coordinating and supervising work: they are also systems for determining goals, coping with conflict and allocating costs as well as benefits. "Organizations perform roles analogous to governments; they may be conceived as *governance systems*" (Walcott & Hult, 1987, p. 112). Some governance tasks may require specialized structures, not associated with ordinary management.

The usefulness of thinking about organizations in governance terms increases with the degree of uncertainty characterizing the decisions to be made. Even choices made in the face of minimal uncertainty imply reliance upon a more broad-based system of formal authority.

Governance theory has also emerged as an alternative to NPM theory. Rhodes (1997b) has argued that NPM is simply one of seven forms of governance. Some now describe *a post-NPM world*, in which NPM alone is no longer sufficient in today's changing environment (Christensen & Laegreid, 2007a,b). Other Europeans propose broadening public management into *public governance* as a way of expanding the focus to include issues of democratic accountability and legitimacy (Kickert, 1997).

Shared governance focuses on participation and decision-making involvement as not the sole responsibility of one (or even a few) top managers but, rather, a collective engagement of individuals working at all levels and in every part of the organization (Alimo-Metcalfe & Alban-Metcalfe, 2006). While, again, no single theoretical definition exists (Gavin et al., 1999), adopted meanings are usually close to that suggested by Geoghegan and Farrington (1995, cited in Scott & Caress, 2005, p. 5): "a system of management and leadership that empowers all staff in decision-making processes". In the health field it is a concept mainly used in literature related to nursing (O'May & Buchan, 1999; Burnhope & Edmonstone, 2003).

Clinical governance emphasizes the importance of quality of care and became popular vocabulary in the United Kingdom, reflected by the 1996 establishment of the *British Journal of Clinical Governance* (in 2003 renamed as *Clinical Governance: An International Journal*). The concept of clinical governance encompasses the interaction between management and physicians, as well as "how to walk the tightrope between public control and professional autonomy" (Burau & Vrangbæk, 2008, p. 365).

1.2.4 The concept of good governance

Several frameworks provide guidance in pursuing *good governance*. In the United States private sector, codes of good organizational governance have existed since January 1978, in the context of charges and counter-charges surrounding corporate takeovers. Since 1989, codes of good governance (primarily at the macro governmental level) have been developed in a number of countries. In the Canadian public sector, for example, a Governance Self-Assessment Checklist was developed (Gill, Flynn & Reissing, 2005). In the United Kingdom, the Chartered Institute of Public Finance and Accountancy (CIPFA, 1994) identified three principles applicable to organizations in the public and private sectors: (1) openness/disclosure of information; (2) integrity/ straightforward dealing and completeness; and (3) accountability/holding individuals responsible for their actions by a clear allocation of responsibilities and defined roles. These codes also reflected general efficiency and legitimacy concerns (Aguilera & Cuervo-Cazurra, 2004).

Beyond the national level, governance codes have also been developed by international organizations. The OECD's 1999 *Principles of corporate governance*, updated in 2004 (OECD, 2004), are among the most authoritative. A 2001 EU White Paper (European Commission, 2001) listed five principles that underpin good governance: (1) openness, (2) participation, (3) accountability, (4) effectiveness and (5) coherence. In the search for good governance in health systems, the function of stewardship has a key role to play (Saltman & Ferroussier-Davis, 2000).

Governing public organizations is understood to differ from governing private enterprises, since ultimate accountability is linked to tax payers rather than stockholders. Public sector governance is also viewed as being more complex than private sector governance, due to less transparent objectives and outcomes of transactions, more widely dispersed power of direction and control, plus an insufficient information environment and conflicting goals – all of which make public organizations relatively prone to poor governance (Kettl, 1993; Hodges, Wright & Keasey, 1996; Lynn, Heinrich & Carolyn, 2001). As applied to hospitals, processes of autonomization, corporatization and privatization have been suggested as ways to influence the interplay between organizational objectives, the supervisory structure and the information environment/market exposure, as well as to protect hospitals by developing measurable goals and establishing professional organizations and performance-based rewards (Preker & Harding, 2003).

1.3 References

Aguilera RV, Cuervo-Cazurra A (2004). Codes of good governance worldwide: what is the trigger? *Organization Studies*, 25(3):415–443.

Alimo-Metcalfe B, Alban-Metcalfe J (2006). More (good) leaders for the public sector. *International Journal of Public Sector Management*, 19(4):293–315.

Alvarez-Rosete A (2007). Modernising policy making. In: Hann A, ed. *Health policy and politics*. Aldershot, Ashgate:41–57.

Andresani G, Ferlie E (2006). Studying governance within the British public sector and without: theoretical and methodological issues. *Public Management Review*, 8:415–431.

Bovaird T, Löffler E (2003). Understanding public management and governance. In: Bovaird T, Löffler E, eds. *Public management and governance.* London, Routledge:3–12.

Braithwaite J et al. (1995). Hospitals: to the next millennium. *International Journal of Health Planning and Management*, 10:87–98.

Burau V, Vrangbæk K (2008). Institutions and non-linear change in governance: reforming the governance of medical performance in Europe. *Journal of Health Organization and Management*, 22(4):350–367.

Burnhope C, Edmonstone J (2003). Feel the fear and do it anyway: the hard business of developing shared governance. *Journal of Nursing Management*, 11:147–157.

Caton D (2000). John Snow's practice of obstetric anaesthesia. *Anaesthesiology*, 92(1):247–252.

Christensen T, Laegreid P (2007a). The whole-of-government approach to public sector reform. *Public Administration Review*, 67(6):1057–1064.

Christensen T, Laegreid P (2007b). *Transcending new public management: the transformation of public sector reforms.* Aldershot, Ashgate.

CIPFA (1994). *Corporate governance in the public services.* London, Chartered Institute of Public Finance and Accountancy.

Degeling P, Erskine J (2009). New models of long-term care and implications for service redesign. In: Rechel B et al., eds. *Investing in hospitals of the future.* Copenhagen, WHO Regional Office for Europe on behalf of the European Observatory on Health Systems and Policies:27–44.

Dixon A et al. (2010). *Patient choice; how patients choose and how providers respond.* London, The King's Fund.

Durán A (2009). Los hospitales del futuro [The hospitals of the future]. *Eidon, Journal of the Institute of Health Sciences*, 29 (Special Issue) (http://www.fcs.es/eidon/eidon29_hospitales_futuro.html, accessed 2 May 2011).

Durán A, Lara JL, van Waveren M (2006). Spain: health system review. *Health Systems in Transition*, 8(4):1–208.

European Commission (2001). *European governance: a white paper.* Brussels, European Commission (http://ec.europa.eu/governance/white_paper/en.pdf, accessed 4 July 2011) (25.7.2001 COM(2001) 428).

Ezzamel M, Reed M (2008). Governance: a code of multiple colours. *Human Relations*, 61(5):597–615.

Fries JF (1980). Aging, natural death and the compression of morbidity. *New England Journal of Medicine*, 303(3):130–135.

Gamble A (2000). Economic governance, In: Pierre J, ed. *Debating governance: authority, steering and democracy*. Oxford, Oxford University Press.

Gavin M et al. (1999). Shared governance: time to consider the cons as well as the pros. *Journal of Nursing Management*, 7(4):193–200.

Geoghegan J, Farrington A (1995). Shared governance: developing a British model. *British Journal of Nursing*, 4(13):780–783.

Gill M, Flynn RJ, Reissing E (2005). The governance self-assessment checklist, an instrument for assessing board effectiveness. *Non-profit management and leadership*, 15(3):271–294.

Greenwood J, Pyper R, Wilson D (2002). *New public administration in Britain*. London, Routledge.

Halpern MT, Yabroff KR (2008). Prevalence of outpatient cancer treatment in the United States: estimates from the Medical Panel Expenditures Survey (MEPS). *Cancer Investigation*, 26(6):647–651.

Hensher M, Edwards N (1999). Hospital provision, activity and productivity in England since the 1980s. *BMJ*, 319(7214):911.

Hodges R, Wright M, Keasey K (1996). Corporate governance in the public services: concepts and issues. *Public Money & Management*, (April–June):7–13.

Hoek H (2007). *Governance & Gezondheidszorg; Private, publieke en professionele invloeden op zorgaanbieders in Nederland [Governance and health care; private, public and professional impact of care providers in the Netherlands]*. Assen, Van Gorcum.

Hood C (1991). A public management for all seasons? *Public Administration*, 69:3–19.

Hood C (2006). The tools of government in the information age. In: Moran M, Rein M, Goodin RE, eds. *The Oxford handbook of political science*. Oxford, Oxford University Press:469–481.

Imison C, Naylor C, Maybin J (2008). *Under one roof. Will polyclinics deliver integrated care?* London, The King's Fund.

Kettl D (1993). Sharing power: public governance and private markets. Washington, DC, Brookings Institution.

Kickert WJM (1997). Public governance in the Netherlands: an alternative to Anglo-American managerialism. *Public Administration*, 75:731–752.

Kjær AM (2004). *Governance*. Cambridge, Polity Press.

Kooiman J (2000). Societal governance: levels, models, and orders of social-political interaction. In: Pierre J, ed. *Debating governance: authority, steering and democracy*. Oxford, Oxford University Press:138–166.

Kuhlmann E, Allsop J, Saks M (2009). Professional governance and public control: a comparison of healthcare in United Kingdom and Germany. *Current Sociology*, 57:511–528.

Lee SYD, Chen WL, Weiner BJ (2004). Communities and hospitals: social capital, community accountability, and service provision in US community hospitals. *Health Services Research*, 39(5):1487–1509.

Lentz EM (1957). Hospital administration – one of a species. *Administrative Science Quarterly*, 1(4):444–463.

Lynn L, Heinrich C, Carolyn J (2001). *Improving governance: a new logic for empirical research*. Washington, DC, Georgetown University Press.

Lynn L, Heinrich C, Hill C (2000). Studying governance and public management: challenges and prospects. *Journal of Public Administration Research and Theory*, 10(2):233–261.

Maarse H, Normand CH (2009). Market competition in European hospital care. In: Rechel B et al., eds. *Investing in hospitals of the future*. Copenhagen, WHO Regional Office for Europe on behalf of the European Observatory on Health Systems and Policies:103–123.

McKee M, Healy J, eds. (2002). *Hospitals in a changing Europe*. Buckingham, Open University Press.

Maybin J (2007). *The reconfiguration of hospital services in England*. London, The King's Fund (http://www.kingsfund.org.uk/publications/briefings/the_reconfiguration.html, accessed 5 September 2010).

Mintzberg H (1983). *Power in and around organizations*. Englewood Cliffs, NJ, Prentice Hall.

Newman J (2001). *Modernising governance. New Labour, policy and society*. London, Sage.

Nolte E, Bain C, McKee M (2006). Chronic diseases as tracer conditions in international benchmarking of health systems: the example of diabetes. *Diabetes Care*, 29:1007–1011.

OECD (2004). *OECD principles of corporate governance*. Paris, Organisation for Economic Co-operation and Development (http://www.oecd.org/dataoecd/32/18/31557724.pdf, accessed 2 May 2011).

OECD (2008). Health Data 2008 [online database]. Paris, Organisation for Economic Co-operation and Development (http://www.oecd.org/departmen t/0,3355,en_2649_34631_1_1_1_1_1,00.html, accessed 5 September 2010).

O'May F, Buchan J (1999). Shared governance: a literature review. *International Journal of Nursing Studies*, 36:281–300.

Or Z et al. (2010). Are health problems systemic? Politics of access and choice under Beveridge and Bismarck systems. *Health Economics Policy and Law*, 5(3):269–293.

Osborne D, Gaebler T (1992). *Reinventing government.* Reading, MA, Addison Wesley.

Peters BG (2004). Back to the centre? Rebuilding the state. In: Gamble A, Wright T, eds. *Restating the state.* London, Blackwell Publishing:130–140.

Pfeffer J (1981). *Power in organizations.* Marshfield, MA, Pitman.

Pierre J (2000). Introduction: understanding governance. In: Pierre J, ed. *Debating governance: authority, steering and democracy.* Oxford, Oxford University Press: 1–12.

Pierre J, Peters BG (2000). *Governance, politics and the state.* Basingstoke, MacMillan Press.

Preker AS, Harding A (2003). *Innovations in health service delivery: the corporatization of public hospitals.* Washington, DC, World Bank.

Rechel B et al., eds. (2009). *Investing in hospitals of the future.* Copenhagen, WHO Regional Office for Europe on behalf of the European Observatory on Health Systems and Policies.

Rhodes RAW (1996). The new governance: governing without government. *Political Studies*, XLIV:652–667.

Rhodes RAW (1997a). Introduction. In: Kickert WJM, Klijn EH, Koppenjan JFM, eds. *Managing complex networks. Strategies for the public sector.* London, Sage:15.

Rhodes RAW (1997b). *Understanding governance: policy networks, governance, reflexivity and accountability.* Buckingham, Open University Press.

Richards D, Smith MJ (2002). *Governance and public policy in the UK.* Oxford, Oxford University Press.

Rodríguez C et al. (2007). Governance, power, and mandated collaboration in an interorganizational network. *Administration & Society*, 39(2):150–193.

Rosenberg CE (1987). *The care of strangers: the rise of America's hospital system.* New York, Basic Books.

Salamon LM, ed. (2002). *The tools of government: a guide to the new governance.* New York, Oxford University Press.

Saltman RB (1987). Management control in a publicly planned health system: a case study from Finland. *Health Policy,* 8(3):283–298.

Saltman RB (1988). National planning for locally controlled health systems: the Finnish experience. *Journal of Health Politics Policy and Law,* 13:27–51.

Saltman RB, Ferroussier-Davis O (2000). The concept of stewardship in health policy. *Bulletin of the World Health Organization,* 78(6):732–739.

Saltman RB, Figueras J (1997). *European health care reform: analysis of current strategies.* Copenhagen, WHO Regional Office for Europe.

Scott L, Caress AL (2005). Shared governance and shared leadership: meeting the challenges of implementation. *Journal of Nursing Management,* 13:4–12.

Shortell S, Kaluzny A (2006). *Health care management: organization design and behavior.* Clifton Park, NY, Thomson Delmar Learning.

Sibbald B, McDonald R, Roland M (2007). Shifting care from hospitals to the community: a review of the evidence on quality and efficiency. *Journal of Health Services Research and Policy,* 12(2):110–117.

Smith PC et al., eds. (2009). *Performance measurement for health system improvement: experiences, challenges and prospects.* Cambridge, Cambridge University Press.

Stoker G (1997). *Public–private partnerships and urban governance.* In: Pierre J, ed. *Public–private partnerships in Europe and the United States.* London, Macmillan:34–51.

The Joint Commission (2008). *Health care at the crossroads: guiding principles for the development of the hospital of the future.* Oakbrook Terrance, IL The Joint Commission (http://www.jointcommission.org/Guiding_Principles_for_The_Development_of_the_Hospital_of_The_Future_/, accessed 2 May 2011).

van Doeveren V (2009). Rethinking the meaning of governance and good governance. Paper presented at *Governing good and governing well: the first global dialogue on ethical and effective governance.* Amsterdam, 28–30 May, 2009.

van Laarhoven H (2008). *The Orbis way of delivering health care.* Presentation delivered at the European Observatory Venice Summer School, 3–8 August, 2008.

Walcott C, Hult KM (1987). Organizing the White House: structure, environment, and organizational governance. *American Journal of Political Science*, 31(1):109–125.

Weiner B, Shortell S, Alexander J (1997). Promoting clinical involvement in hospital quality improvement efforts: the effects of top management, board, and physician leadership. *Health Services Research*, 32(4):491–510.

WHO Regional Office for Europe (2010). European Health for All database (HFA-DB) [online database]. Copenhagen, WHO Regional Office for Europe (http://data.euro.who.int/hfadb/, accessed 10 March 2010).

Wilson T, Buck D, Ham C (2005). Rising to the challenge: will the NHS support people with long-term conditions? (Review). *BMJ*, 330(7492): 657–661.

Winblad U, Ringard A (2009). Meeting rising public expectations: the changing role of patients and citizens. In: Magnussen J, Vrangbaek K, Saltman RB, eds. *Nordic health care systems: recent reforms and current policy challenges*. Maidenhead, Open University Press:126–150.

World Bank (1989). *From crisis to sustainable development: Africa's long-term perspective*. Washington, DC, World Bank.

Zito A, Radaelli C, Jordan A, eds. (2003). Introduction to the symposium on new policy instruments in the European Union. *Public Administration*, 81(3):509–511.

Chapter 2

A framework for assessing hospital governance

Antonio Durán, Richard B. Saltman and Hans F.W. Dubois

This chapter develops a conceptual framework and a set of criteria for the governance of public hospitals. After a short discussion of recent efforts to establish innovative new hospital governance strategies, it describes a set of criteria for use in assessing the governance process for publicly owned hospitals. The criteria presented are functional in nature, focusing primarily on activities that can be used in assessing the meso institutional level of governance.

2.1 Innovative arrangements in hospital governance

In response to the wide range of institutional, political and fiscal pressures detailed in Chapter 1, health care systems across Europe began to re-examine their steering methods for hospitals. Traditionally, in Europe as elsewhere, public hospitals had been operated according to a strict command-and-control model, with a government-based administration that implemented decisions made by "the owners" – municipal, county, regional and/or national government(s) – depending on the country. As noted earlier, hospital administrators were typically political appointees, directly answerable to political bodies, and serving at their sufferance. Among the numerous dilemmas associated with this type of direct bureaucratic control was the inability to separate local operational decisions inside institutions from the overall policy responsibility of senior politicians. Aneurin Bevan, the British Minister of Health who was instrumental in designing the initial 1948 structure of the National Health

Service (NHS), famously contended that "when a bedpan falls in Tredegar, its sound should echo in the halls of Westminister". While this direct administrative responsibility led to clear lines of political accountability, it established a centralized, bureaucratic model of policy-making and management (that is, of what we now call governance) which severely tied the hands of individual institutional administrators as well as (often) those of the institution's medical staff. In some countries, it led to remarkable situations, such as that witnessed by one author[5] in Spain in 1989, when the Director of the National School of Public Health – a major national policy post – was called out of a major ministerial policy conference at the Ministry of Health and Consumer Affairs in Madrid in order to deal with a personnel crisis that had arisen that morning in one of Madrid's hospitals.

Reform responses to this traditional type of centralized political control have included introducing different levels of institutional autonomy and at least a moderate degree of internal and external market incentives. An increasing number of publicly owned hospitals have been restructured in a broad spectrum of configurations, including exposing service provision to market-like pressures, designing and implementing accountability mechanisms, and transferring some decision-making control to provider organizations. Overall, as part of the developmental process, the boundaries between the public and private sectors in European health care systems have become increasingly blurred (Saltman, 2003).

The ongoing structural shift towards more autonomous models of public hospitals reflects two decades of debate in Europe. Theoretical models that called for the introduction of a "planned market" based on "public competition" among publicly owned and operated hospitals (Saltman & von Otter, 1987), the creation of a new "internal market" in the hospital sector (Enthoven, 1985), or the introduction of a "quasi-market" (Le Grand & Bartlett, 1993) laid the groundwork for major change. Organizational changes began as early as January 1988 in Stockholm County in Sweden (Bruce & Jönsson, 1996) and, in England – following the publication in January 1989 of Margaret Thatcher's White Paper *Working for patients* – in the subsequent introduction in April 1991 of the first version of "Self-governing Trusts" for 57 NHS hospitals (Klein, 1995). Politically important issues of greater efficiency in service production and delivery – along with growing patient demands for more timely access, higher quality services and choice over where and from whom they received their medical care – combined to produce a wide range of new governance strategies in tax-funded health care systems across Europe.

---

5   R.B. Saltman.

Since these initial pioneering efforts, public hospitals in countries in both western and central Europe have become (to varying degrees) quasi-independently operated institutions – what have been termed "public firms" (Saltman & von Otter, 1992a,b) – described as having been through a process of "autonomization and corporatization" (Preker & Harding, 2003). Such organizations are public, to varying degrees, depending on their ownership, funding and control structures, and in many cases they have mimicked private companies by introducing effective incentive systems. Other important developments have included many public hospitals acquiring their own Boards (of Trustees or Supervisors); senior managers (in northern European models) becoming non-political professionals hired on short-term contracts, which need not be renewed; doctors and nurses being hired (and fired) on short-term contracts (sometimes under private law) by the hospital itself; operating surpluses being rolled over for use by the hospital in the next budget year; and capital (in some countries) being raised through the private sector by the hospital itself. The range of detailed models is considerable, involving different governance approaches, and with a level of variation signalled by the notably different terms used for public hospitals in these newly emerging models:

- "self-governing trusts" and "foundation trusts" (United Kingdom);
- "joint-stock companies" and "foundations" (Estonia);
- 'limited liability companies" and "joint-stock companies" (Czech Republic)
- "public-stock corporations" (Sweden);
- "state enterprises" (Norway);
- "public enterprise entity hospitals" (PEEHs, Portugal); and
- "public healthcare companies" (*Empresa Pública Sanitaria*), "public healthcare foundations" (*Fundacións Pública Sanitaria*), "consortia" (*Consorcio*), "foundations" (*Fundacións*) and "administrative concessions" (*Concesión Administrativa*) (Spain).

While each of the above arrangements gives public hospitals more independent decision-making autonomy than they had as directly administered public institutions, the specific mix and impact of these new capacities differs considerably between models.

Assessment of the new role and responsibilities of public hospitals, or of the processes and tools devised to better govern them, needs to accommodate the crucial impact that both national context and culture have on how these new models are structured, on their behaviour when implemented, and on the likelihood of achieving their intended policy objectives (Saltman, in press).

Context is a wide-ranging concept that extends from geographic conditions in a country's physical layout (which, for example, affects the location and size of its hospital configuration), to its workforce capacities (a shortage of nurses will alter policy options for expanded outpatient services) and to the country's overall fiscal condition (large deficits preclude increases in staff salaries).

Culture, while more elusive, reflects the social norms and values that influence political and social decisions relating to acceptable institutional activity and behaviour (Hofstede, 1980, 1991). While cultural anthropologists disparage the concept of a "national culture" as static and simplistic (Benhabib, 2002), national policy-makers nonetheless differ in the decisions they make about their health sectors, and in particular regarding the degrees of operating freedom that they are in practice willing to confer on their public hospitals, based on their sense of the social expectations of the citizenry as a whole (Saltman & Bergman, 2005). As the evidence from the case studies in this volume demonstrates, the level of operating autonomy that an Estonian or Czech Minister of Health considers appropriate for a hospital is quite different to the level of autonomy that a Spanish or Norwegian politician believes is normatively acceptable for one of their public hospitals. Moreover, the degree of fiscal pressure that a government faces will often directly translate into the type of measures that it imposes on all public agencies under its purview, including public hospitals.

The above-mentioned considerations raise a number of issues concerning the scope, character and usefulness of the various ongoing public hospital governance initiatives. To move from generalities to specifics, however, these concepts need to be translated into meaningful organizational dimensions (and relevant research questions) that reflect the particular circumstances and characteristics which influence the decision-making process within individual countries.

2.2 Framework for operationalizing hospital governance

Following on from the Introduction, this section builds a framework of functional concepts for assessing meso-level "hospital governance" models in Europe, setting out specifications for the key relationships between the main variables involved. The general definition of hospital governance used in this study – from which this more specific meso-level framework is derived – is as follows:

> A set of processes and tools related to decision-making in steering the totality of institutional activity, influencing most major aspects of organizational behaviour and recognizing the complex relationships between multiple stakeholders. Its scope ranges from normative values (equity, ethics) to access, quality, patient responsiveness, and patient safety dimensions. It also incorporates political, financial, managerial as well as daily operational issues.

As used in this volume, therefore, the term "hospital governance" emphasizes a set of discrete processes and tools, rather than just one or more specific location or organization at which or in which these processes or tools are utilized. Moreover, this definition highlights that the act of governance reflects a variety of institutional elements and/or shareholders, at macro (national), meso (whole-institutional) and micro (operational management) levels. In practice, many players can participate separately or simultaneously in the governance process: national, regional or local government, the Supervisory Board, the Management (or Executive) Board, senior management staff, physician heads of clinical departments, the medical staff organization, and also various types of patient groups, all of which create a complex mosaic of decision-making relationships among and between different actors, both within and beyond the hospital walls. Collectively, they deal with the wide range of activities listed in the definition, such that outcomes can be affected by interventions of various oversight organizations focusing on clinical quality, patient safety, staff qualifications, accreditation and financial accounting. Notably, this definition of hospital governance reflects the complex multidimensionality of public policy decision-making in the first decade of the 21st century, as detailed in the Introduction and Chapter 1.

The next step involves framing the objective of specifically meso-level public hospital governance – that is, the goal of decisions made in response to the question "*what* are hospital level 'governors' expected to achieve?" The answer is in practical terms rather straightforward: improve the operation of the hospital, as reflected in better clinical, financial and patient satisfaction outcomes. Meso-level hospital governance should ensure high levels of service quality and of responsiveness to patients, while efficiently maximizing the return from available resources within a given regulatory framework.

In practice, of course, it is difficult in technical terms to measure the relationships that exist between governance and performance. In each country, hospitals pursue objectives along courses of action that are strongly related to their own national history, culture and context, often barely comparable one to another, reflecting the set of previous policy choices (Oliver & Mossialos, 2005). Even in terms of capital investment, the effort to assess hospitals using common metrics is in its infancy (Rechel et al., 2009).

While useful quantitative performance measures are currently being developed (Smith et al., 2010), they are still at an early stage of refinement. Moreover, despite recent initial conclusions taken from very large hospital samples (Bloom et al., 2010), specific institutional-level linkage of meso-level governance strategies to clinical, financial and patient-related outcomes remains highly qualitative in nature.

When looking at this qualitative linkage between meso-level hospital governance decisions and institutional outcomes, the eight country case studies in this volume reinforce the theoretical assumption that hospital autonomy matters. Autonomy is a crucial attribute of institutional governance in the current economic and political context, as detailed in Chapter 1, which requires the hospital to adopt innovative new approaches, not in its objectives but rather in how those objectives are achieved. While the link between hospital autonomy and performance is not a direct consequence of the changing relationship between state and society, the central policy objective must be to ensure that publicly operated hospitals have the necessary degrees of freedom to confront contemporary challenges. Hence, the central variable examined in the eight country case studies becomes the substantial degree of hospital autonomy.

Drawing from this concept of institutional autonomy, the hospitals in the eight countries selected for case studies fall into only two of the four general types of hospital that currently can be found across Europe. These four general types are:

1. regular public hospitals with direct political management, mostly existing in tax-funded systems (Finland, much of Sweden, Ireland, the former Yugoslav Republic of Macedonia) but also some – especially tertiary care university hospitals – in social health insurance (SHI)-funded systems (France, Germany, Switzerland);

2. semi-autonomous public hospitals with various degrees of independent decision-making, existing in tax-funded systems of various types (Norway, Estonia, England; some hospitals in Spain – Andalucía, Balearic Islands, Catalonia, Madrid, Murcia and Valencia – as well as in Portugal; several northern regions of Italy; Israel; and the Czech Republic);

3. non-profit-making private hospitals – typically with religious or community missions and boards, which mostly receive funding through public channels, particularly in SHI systems (Netherlands, Germany, Switzerland), but also in small numbers in some tax-funded systems (England, Sweden);

4. profit-making private hospitals – typically small clinics that are often started by physicians, particularly in countries with SHI systems (France, Germany, Switzerland), but also a small number in some tax-funded countries (Denmark, Norway).

The study focuses on types 2 and 3 in the continuum of governance models, precisely because this is where recent reforms of public hospitals based on semi-autonomous strategies have been introduced. Categories 2 and 3 represent the efforts to date to rethink public hospital governance in Europe. While the other two categories of hospitals – directly managed public as well as profit-making hospitals – have undergone reforms, they have not pursued equivalently innovative governance strategies. Countries in which the need to act more "autonomously" has crystallized can provide useful examples of new styles of meso-level public hospital governance. Semi-autonomous models of public hospitals – as noted in the Introduction – are the subject of keen interest among national policy-makers in a number of European countries, which either still have predominantly directly managed public hospitals or which seek to compare their own semi-autonomous public model with those introduced in other countries. In addition, the relevance of private non-profit-making hospitals as conceptual end-points for how far this process of autonomy can extend (within the context of remaining socially and politically accountable) explains the inclusion of the Netherlands and, to a lesser extent, the Czech Republic and Estonia. This emphasis on the degree of hospital autonomy as the key variable also informs the choice of the four factors used to assess meso-level hospital governance in the study. These four aspects are explained here.

1. *Institutional dimension.* Who are you? What are your credentials? To what are you entitled? Are you recognized as "different and special", or not?

2. *Financing dimension.* What freedom do you have to handle your resources? From where do you get your money? How do you cope with your capital and revenue needs? What is your process for managing investments and running costs?

3. *Accountability dimension.* On behalf of whom are you acting? To whom do you report? What kind of organizational structure do you have in that context? Who is involved in your decision-making processes?

4. *Correspondence between responsibility and decision-making capacity.* Can you honour your promises? Are you able to negotiate and reach agreements with others? How do you adjust to contingencies? How transparent are your day-to-day operating decisions?

Framed in more detailed terms, the variables involved are as follows.

a. *Institutional arrangements*:
   - legal form and objectives (social, political)
   - room for decisions (clinical services, locations, incentives/sanctions)
   - relations with stakeholders: role of professional organizations, unions.

b. *Financial arrangements*:
   - capital investment (sources, constraints, conditions)
   - adjusting capital and operational expenses: additional sources, loans
   - ability to retain surpluses and incur debt.

c. *Accountability arrangements*:
- supervisory Board (role, size, composition, appointments)
- citizen and patient involvement and participation
- reporting obligations (completeness, transparency and timing).

d. *Decision-making capacity versus responsibility*:
- room to adjust to unexpected trends/freedom from political interference
- power sharing with clinicians (clinical trials, partnerships including equipment, hiring and firing)
- flexibility in internal monitoring, follow-up and evaluation.

Clearly categories a, b and c address decision-making by the hospital stakeholders based on broad objectives and strategies and align with what could be called *strategic governance*, related to global institutional, financial and accountability arrangements. While some of these arrangements are typically defined by the state at the macro level, others are defined or influenced by meso-level hospital decisions. Category d refers to the ability to implement the decisions of the hospital board and other meso-level governance structures in searching for innovative approaches throughout the day-to-day life of the hospital, and could be described as *operational governance*.

Section 2.3 presents a more elaborated discussion of these four categories within the study's framework and how they relate to the hospital sector generally.

2.3 Exploring the study's key variables in detail

Institutional arrangements are a central aspect of hospital governance, of which a key element is the legal form that the hospital takes. Foundations, corporatized public companies, public entities with delegated management and other "new" types of institution typically include mechanisms and tools to help hospitals strive for a desired set of objectives (social, political, etc.) and to preserve public values in a market-oriented model. Also, stakeholders (unions, professional organizations, patient organizations, citizen groups) may participate in decisions regarding clinical services, locations, incentives/sanctions, and so on. Hospital staff involvement can vary widely and may be formalized through board membership, regular consultation or informal dialogue (see, for example, Dubois, 2002; Gautam, 2005). Typically, traditional political, employee union and physician actors that had exercised considerable influence over publicly operated institutions in the past lose much of their authority in these new decision-making models (Saltman & von Otter, 1987).

These structural developments reflect a range of prior and ongoing efforts to introduce organizational change. NPM reforms have often sought to weaken the managerial role of physicians by opening up institutional management positions to professional managers who may be non-clinicians (Ferlie & Fitzgerald, 2000; Scott et al., 2000; Dent, 2003). According to some evaluators, however, these reforms have not always led to major changes in the administrative–professional relationship (Kitchener, 1999, for the United Kingdom; Jespersen, Nielsen & Sognstrup, 2002, for Denmark).

Financial arrangements are a second critical element of meso-level hospital governance. Both capital and operating budgets have been the focus of recent reforms. Although hospital capital decisions are still predominantly made in the public domain and are dominated by centralized models (Ettelt et al., 2008), recent changes in how day-to-day operating funds are allocated have tended to reflect a more market-oriented approach (relating hospital funding to performance; more stringent public procurement procedures; growth of the profit-making market segment; and initiatives to shorten waiting times by inviting the private sector to compete for public funding in hospital care).

In countries with tax-funded health systems, it is rarely electorally or socially acceptable to discuss selling off publicly built and publicly capitalized institutions, or otherwise to put at risk universal access to those institutions' services. Moreover, publicly owned hospitals in Europe typically operate in a tightly controlled environment in which they are not allowed to make capital investment plans or bear financial risks, but rather depend on political decisions for approval. Yet, public hospitals increasingly need considerable autonomy in their day-to-day operating decisions if they are to respond to the multiple demands relating to patient needs, professional preferences and the concerns of other stakeholders. This decision-making environment makes it valuable also to determine what scope reform models may give hospitals in terms of handling capital investment themselves (sources, constraints, conditions) and adjusting their operating expenses, finding additional sources of funds and arranging loans.

In the non-profit-making hospitals in the Netherlands, by contrast, price competition for operating income is increasingly complemented by "yardstick competition", using maximum tariffs centrally set by the Dutch Health Care Authority for specific hospital services, thereby allowing efficient hospitals and independent treatment centres (ITCs) to retain surplus revenue (Maarse & Normand, 2009). In England, the creation of Foundation Trusts has also given hospitals more control over assets, the ability to raise a certain amount of financial resources, and more accountability (see Chapter 6). The situation could become more complex if hospitals were allowed to attract investment partners, property agencies or other private companies in new partnerships, similar to the Private Finance Initiative (PFI) introduced in the United Kingdom, or the Alzira Hospital model in Spain (see Chapter 12).

A consistent trend in European hospitals is to move away from global budgets towards case-mix-based funding (payment by activity), so that public and private commissioning agencies/purchasers can assess the volume and quality of hospital production. This calls for more time and effort to be spent on the recording, coding and detailed costing of activities, a precondition for effective internal market arrangements. Much is yet to be achieved before hospitals learn to fully navigate the new funding schemes, especially in the absence of more refined measurement tools (Durán et al., 2004). Accurately predicting how the relationship with funding agencies may evolve will be more critical for innovative hospitals than it will be for other non-budgetary entities, as they will have to cope with a higher degree of uncertainty. Market contract terms, for example, are rather clear compared with how contracts with funding agencies reward cost control or quality of care – to name two objectives on which there is remarkably little reliable information. Ensuring proper follow-up to learn from experience will be crucial.

A related financing issue is that in some countries public hospitals pay their CEOs less, compared with private hospitals, with consequent selection and incentive problems, poor operating performance and high turnover of board members (Preyra & Pink, 2001; Eldenburg et al., 2004). NHS Trusts in England and Wales also pay less to their external auditors than their private sector counterparts (Clatworthy, Mellett & Peel, 2008), probably as a consequence of the Trusts being more heavily regulated. Moreover, receiving government funding shifts energy away from certain activities (that is, traditional board functions such as fund raising) towards others, such as financial monitoring and advocacy (O'Regan & Oster, 2002).

Accountability arrangements are a third important aspect of meso-level hospital governance. These can be decisive within the public realm, in which different hospital actors are held accountable for their actions in a context of increased autonomy, improved "intelligence" and more robust information systems. Political bodies and authorities also play a complex role within new hospital governance models. On the one hand, innovative models are designed to push back against and/or restrain the interference of local and regional political actors in decision-making by publicly owned and operated hospitals. The argument in favour of creating political firewalls has been exhaustively documented since the late 1980s.[6] From the other side of the structural coin, in most countries with publicly owned hospitals, some ultimate form of accountability/political supervision is viewed as being essential.

---

6 See, for example, Bartlett et al., 1994; Saltman & von Otter, 1995; Jerome-Forget, White & Wiener, 1995; Ranade, 1998; Powell & Wesson, 1999; European Observatory on Health Systems and Policies volumes, including Mossialos et al., 2002; Saltman, Busse & Mossialos, 2002; Figueras, Robinson & Jakubowski, 2005.

In this context of complex decisions and multiple agents, governance of public hospitals requires that actors are accountable for processes and procedures as much as for outcomes and financial compliance (Bovens, 2006). The challenge is how to establish "clear loci of responsibility, enough information and appropriate sanctions" (Tuohy, 2003, p. 196). Moreover, accountability has a number of dimensions – financial, performance and political/democratic (Brinkerhoff, 2004) – that make it more complicated than traditional management. Innovative hospital governance models seek to reduce direct political accountability of elected political authorities for these hospitals' day-to-day clinical and financial decisions. The long-term importance of maintaining overall accountability for social responsibility in health systems has been set out in several spirited defences of the social and political role of publicly owned and operated hospitals (Dahlgren, 1994; Pollock, 2004).

The roles and functions of the Supervisory Board are directly related topics, along with citizen participation and patient involvement (Lee et al., 2008). Different emphasis is placed on Boards of Directors in different groups of hospitals, in terms of their functions – for example, mission and strategy setting, advisory role to management, performance evaluation, oversight and control (Lee et al., 2008). The function and composition of such boards have been identified as important factors in hospitals obtaining community support and attracting resources from the environment (Pfeffer, 1973, 1981). The role of the Board of Directors of a hospital is likely to vary with a number of factors – size of budget; proportion of capital funds obtained from private donations; importance of fund raising as a board function and importance of selecting board members for their ability to raise money, influence in the local community and whether the hospital is private, non-profit-making or has a religious affiliation.

Contextual factors such as size can influence the uncertainties faced by the hospital, which, in turn, affects the characteristics of administrators (Pfeffer & Salancik, 1977). Empirical evidence regarding the impact of board characteristics is mixed, reflecting such factors as staff structure and composition (Succi & Alexander, 1999), interrelationships with environment and strategy (Hambrick, 1981) and country context-dependent differences in mechanisms (Gerowitz et al., 1996). A social network perspective in assessing board composition suggests that who sits on the hospital board, how the members are selected, and how many members it has disclose much about the board's character (Johnson, Nielsen & Sognstrup, 1996; Lynall, Golden & Hillman, 2003). Board members' age, gender, tenure, occupational background, educational background, the diversity of and change in those characteristics, the size of the board, and functional arrangements (term limits, meeting frequency, formal functions) have all been identified as relevant endogenous and explanatory governance variables – although evidence is mixed and contradictory at times (Alexander, Weiner & Bogue, 2001). Board diversity can inhibit strategic change (Goodstein, Gautam & Boeker, 1994) and boards with low turnover pay excessive compensation to their CEOs – which suggests that managerial entrenchment, rather than efficient contracting, creates this result (Cahan, Chua & Nyamori, 2005).

There is evidence that strategic change may be affected by board demography and processes, and that these effects seem to manifest most strongly in situations in which boards are more powerful (Golden & Zajac, 2001). Business executives, physicians and hospital executives as board members provide links to different community segments. Depth of innovation has also been shown to be related to the proportion of involved members – although the overall level of innovation seemed to depend on dynamic, social group processes (West & Anderson, 1996). Hospitals often attempt to cope with changes in potential sources of uncertainty by changing the composition of their boards (Boeker & Goodstein, 1991).

"Does the hospital board need a doctor?" is a frequent question that arises (Molinari et al., 1995). Governmental or hospital rules mandating hospitals to have physicians on their boards are not uncommon – NHS Trust boards in England are required to include at least one medical director and a director of nursing (Ferlie, Ashburner & Fitzgerald, 1995). However, one researcher concluded that two decades of empirical investigation of this issue had been broadly inconclusive (Denis, 2001).

Including citizens on hospital boards as a form of citizen involvement is only likely to influence hospital behaviour when there is an active political culture (Lee, Chen & Weiner, 2004), but it does not guarantee public interest representation, since those citizens involved may champion personal concerns (Cagle, Martinez & Richardson, 1999) or may not represent normal service users (Hayllar, 1999). Public participation might also be achieved by including locally – and democratically – appointed non-executive board members as an interface with the local community, or through representative committees such as those found in New Zealand and Sweden (Ham, 1994). Opening board meetings to the public is another way to improve community involvement, although such meetings can have a somewhat chilling effect on the candidness of discussion and prevent quick action if advanced announcements are required – an important distinction between short-term and long-term accountability (Zablocki, 2007). In addition, the number of members of the public who actually attend such meetings can be disappointing (Ferlie, Fitzgerald & Ashburner, 1996).

Finally, *decision-making capacity versus responsibility* is a central dimension for the structure of hospital governance. This is the acid test of autonomy from a governance perspective, due to its importance in setting up new power relationships. Since "governance" as a concept involves a special emphasis on implementation (Pierre & Peters, 2000), the vital quandary relates to where to draw the line between high-level decisions (macro level) and decision processes that – for reasons of efficiency, effectiveness, quality and responsiveness – ought to be separated from direct political scrutiny and control. To what extent the high-level goals and politics of recent health system reforms give hospitals sufficient room to adjust to unexpected trends in practice, free from undue political interference at ground level, is a major indicator of hospital autonomy.

Although all four strategic issues outlined here are important for public hospital governance,[7] there has been little comparative study of what emerging forms of hospital semi-autonomy mean *in practice*, in terms of real decision and control at ground level. Understanding decisions in terms of their broader public and social interest requires political bodies – and thus those who staff them, such as elected politicians – to allow hospital directors to review and/or reverse decisions made at the institutional level, without breaking the planning rationality and still being held accountable at a later stage. These decisions may be linked to power-sharing arrangements with clinicians and other staff (partnerships, purchase of equipment, adjustments to policies relating to hiring and firing, clinical trials, etc.). Governance reforms that do more in terms of giving an appropriate role to health professionals have generally fallen short (Ham, 2003). The limited impacts of health care reforms stems in part from their limited effects on clinical practice. There are many factors that influence decisions by health professionals and patients (Fishbein et al., 2001; Wensing et al., 2001; Cochrane, Olson & Murray, 2007) and policies introduced by health care reformers need to compete with these concerns. Thus, no single approach or intervention is likely to be sufficient (Oxman et al., 2008, pp. 17–18).

Flexibility in internal monitoring, follow-up and evaluation is a necessary condition of improving results. Appropriate standards of governance require adequate operational information flows in many directions – including from the bottom to the top – as a precondition not only to preclude gaming behaviour and "service creep" (that is, being classified as more complex so as to attract higher fees) (Nassiri & Rochaix, 2006), but also to promote quality and efficiency of hospital care based on informed decision-making by providers. A United Kingdom study (Bloom et al., 2010) argues that public hospitals have significantly worse management practices than private hospitals, although management ratings among publicly owned hospitals are relatively high for

---

7   See, for example, van Doorslaer et al., 2000; Berwick, 2003; Saltman, Figueras & Busse, 2004; Porter & Teisberg, 2004.

Foundation Trusts (hospitals with greater autonomy from government), for larger hospitals, and in settings in which managers have more clinical expertise.

2.4 References

Alexander JA, Weiner BJ, Bogue RJ (2001). Changes in the structure, composition and activity of hospital governing boards, 1989–1997: evidence from two national surveys. *Milbank Quarterly*, 79(2):253–279.

Bartlett W et al. (1994). *Quasi-markets in the welfare state*. Bristol, University of Bristol SAUS Publications.

Benhabib S (2002). *The claims of culture: equality and diversity in the global era*. Princeton, NJ, Princeton University Press.

Berwick DM (2003). Disseminating innovations in health care. *Journal of the American Medical Association*, 289:1969–1975.

Bloom N et al. (2010). *Why good practices really matter in healthcare*. London, VoxEU.org, Centre for Economic Policy and Research (http://www.voxeu.org/index.php?q=node/5939, accessed 2 May 2011).

Boeker W, Goodstein J (1991). Organizational performance and adaptation: effects of environment and performance on changes in board composition. *Academy of Management Journal*, 34(4):805–826.

Bovens M (2006). Analysing and assessing public accountability. A conceptual framework. *European Governance Papers (EUROGOV)*, No. C-06-01 (http://www.connex-network.org/eurogov/pdf/egp-connex-C-06-01.pdf, accessed 2 May 2011).

Brinkerhoff DW (2004). Accountability and health systems: toward conceptual clarity and policy relevance. *Health Policy and Planning*, 19(6):371–379.

Bruce A, Jönsson E (1996). *Competition in the provision of health care: the experience of the US, Sweden and Britain*. Aldershot, Arena.

Cagle MC, Martinez JM, Richardson WD (1999). Privatizing professional licensing boards: self-governance or self-interest? *Administration & Society*, 30:734–770.

Cahan SF, Chua F, Nyamori RO (2005). Board structure and executive compensation in the public sector: New Zealand evidence. *Financial Accountability & Management*, 21(4):437–465.

Clatworthy MA, Mellett HJ, Peel MJ (2008). Changes in NHS Trust audit and non-audit fees. *Public Money & Management*, 28(4):199–205.

Cochrane LJ, Olson CA, Murray S (2007). Gaps between knowing and doing: understanding and assessing the barriers to optimal health care. *Journal of Continuing Education in the Health Professions*, 27:94–102.

Dahlgren G (1994). *Framtidens Sjukvardsmarknarder – vinnare och förlorare? [Health care markets of the future – winners and losers?]*. Stockholm, Natur och Kultur.

Denis DK (2001). Twenty-five years of corporate governance research ... and counting. *Review of Financial Economics*, 10:191–212.

Dent M (2003). *Remodelling hospitals and health professions in Europe: medicine, nursing and the state*. Basingstoke, Palgrave Macmillan.

Dubois HFW (2002). Harmonization of the European vaccination policy and the role TQM and reengineering could play. *Quality Management in Health Care*, 10(2):47–57.

Durán A et al. (2004). Health care contracts. In: Figueras J, Robinson R, Jakubowski E, eds. *Purchasing to improve health systems performance*. Buckingham, Open University Press:187–214.

Eldenburg L et al. (2004). Governance, performance objectives and organizational form: evidence from hospitals. *Journal of Corporate Finance*, 10:527–548.

Enthoven A (1985). *Reflections on the NHS*. London, Nuffield Trust.

Ettelt S et al. (2008). *Capacity planning in health care: a review of the international experience*. Copenhagen, WHO Regional Office for Europe on behalf of the European Observatory on Health Systems and Policies (Policy Brief, No. 13).

Ferlie E, Fitzgerald LF (2000). Professionals: back to the future? *Human Relations*, 53(5):713–739.

Ferlie E, Ashburner L, Fitzgerald LF (1995). Corporate governance and the public sector: some issues and evidence from the NHS. *Public Administration*, 73:375–392.

Ferlie E, Fitzgerald LF, Ashburner L (1996). Corporate governance in the post-1990 NHS: the role of the board. *Public Money & Management*, 16:15–21.

Figueras J, Robinson R, Jakubowski E, eds. (2005). *Purchasing to improve health systems performance*. Maidenhead, Open University Press.

Fishbein M et al. (2001). Factors influencing behavior and behavior change, In: Baum A, Revenson TA, Singer JE, eds. *Handbook of health psychology*. Mahwah, NJ, Lawrence Erlbaum:3–17.

Gautam KS (2005). A call for board leadership on quality in hospitals. *Quality Management in Health Care*, 14(1):18–30.

Gerowitz MB et al. (1996). Top management culture and performance in Canadian, UK and US hospitals. *Health Service Management Research*, 9(2): 69–78.

Golden BR, Zajac EJ (2001). When will boards influence strategy? Inclination x power = strategic change. *Strategic Management Journal*, 22(12):1087–1111.

Goodstein J, Gautam K, Boeker W (1994). The effects of board size and diversity on strategic change. *Strategic Management Journal*, 15(3):241–250.

Ham C (1994). When health care goes on the ration. *The Guardian*, 9 November 1994.

Ham C (2003). Improving the performance of health services: the role of clinical leadership. *Lancet*, 361:1978–1980.

Hambrick DC (1981). Environment, strategy, and power within top management teams. *Administrative Science Quarterly*, 26(2):253–275.

Hayllar MR (1999). Reforms to enhance accountability and citizen involvement: a case study of the Hong Kong hospital authority. *International Journal of Public Administration*, 22(3&4):461–498.

Hofstede G (1980). *Culture's consequences*. Beverly Hills, CA, Sage.

Hofstede G (1991). *Cultures and organizations*. London, Harper Collins Business.

Jerome-Forget M, White J, Wiener JM, eds. (1995). *Health care reform through internal markets: experience and proposals*. Washington, DC, Brookings Institution.

Jespersen PK, Nielsen L, Sognstrup H (2002). Professions, institutional dynamics, and new public management in the Danish hospital field. *International Journal of Public Administration*, 25(12):1555–1574.

Johnson PK, Nielsen LLM, Sognstrup H (1996). Professions, institutional dynamics, and new public management in the Danish hospital field. *International Journal of Public Administration*, 25(12):1555–1574.

Kitchener M (1999). All fur coat and no knickers – contemporary organizational change in United Kingdom hospitals. In: Brock D, Powell M, Hinings CR, eds. *Restructuring the professional organization*. London, Routledge:183–199.

Klein R (1995). Big bang health reform: does it work? The case of Britain's 1991 National Health Service reforms. *Milbank Quarterly*, 73(3):299–338.

Lee SYD, Chen WL, Weiner BJ (2004). Communities and hospitals: social capital, community accountability, and service provision in US community hospitals. *Health Services Research*, 39(5):1487–1509.

Lee SYD et al. (2008). An empirical taxonomy of hospital governing board roles. *Health Services Research*, 43(4):1223–1243.

Le Grand J, Bartlett W, eds. (1993). *Quasi-markets and social policy*. Basingstoke, MacMillan Press.

Lynall MD, Golden BR, Hillman A (2003). Board composition from adolescence to maturity: a multitheoretic view. *Academy of Management Review*, 28(3):416–431.

Maarse H, Normand CH (2009). Market competition in European hospital care. In: Rechel B et al., eds. *Investing in hospitals of the future*. Copenhagen, WHO Regional Office for Europe on behalf of the European Observatory on Health Systems and Policies:103–123.

Molinari C et al. (1995). Does the hospital board need a doctor? The influence of physician board participation on hospital financial performance. *Medical Care*, 33(2):170–185.

Mossialos E et al. (2002). *Funding health care: options for Europe*. Buckingham, Open University Press.

Nassiri A, Rochaix L (2006). Revisiting physicians' financial incentives in Quebec: a panel system approach. *Health Economics*, 15(1):49–64.

Oliver AJ, Mossialos EA (2005). European health systems reform: looking backward to see forward. *Journal of Health Politics, Policy and Law*, 30(1–2): 7–28.

O'Regan K, Oster S (2002). Does government funding alter non-profit governance? Evidence from New York City non-profit contractors. *Journal of Policy Analysis and Management*, 21(3):359–379.

Oxman AD et al. (2008). *Integrated health care for people with chronic conditions. A Policy Brief*. Oslo, Norwegian Knowledge Centre for the Health Services.

Pfeffer J (1973). Size, composition, and function of hospital boards of directors: a study of organization–environment linkage. *Administrative Science Quarterly*, 18(3):349–364.

Pfeffer J (1981). *Power in organizations*. Marshfield, MA, Pitman.

Pfeffer J, Salancik GR (1977). Organizational context and the characteristics and tenure of hospital administrators. *Academy of Management Journal*, 20(1):74–88.

Pierre J, Peters BG (2000). *Governance, politics and the state*. Basingstoke, MacMillan Press.

Pollock A (2004). *NHS plc: the privatisation of our health care*. London, Verso.

Porter ME, Teisberg EO (2004). Redefining competition in health care. *Harvard Business Review*, 82(6):64–76.

Powell FD, Wessen AF, eds. (1999). *Health care systems in transition: an international perspective*. London, Sage.

Preker AS, Harding A (2003). *Innovations in health service delivery: the corporatization of public hospitals*. Washington, DC, World Bank.

Preyra C, Pink G (2001). Balancing incentives in the compensation contracts of non-profit hospital CEOs. *Journal of Health Economics*, 20(4):509–525.

Ranade W, ed. (1998). *Markets and health care: a comparative analysis*. London, Longman.

Rechel et al., eds. (2009). *Investing in hospitals of the future*. Copenhagen, WHO Regional Office for Europe on behalf of the European Observatory on Health Systems and Policies.

Saltman RB (2003). The melting public–private boundary in European health care systems. *European Journal of Public Health*, 13(1):24–29.

Saltman RB (in press). Context, culture and the practical limits of health sector accountability. In: Israeli A, Rosen B, Shortell S, eds. *Accountability and responsibility in health care*. London, World Scientific Publishers.

Saltman RB, Bergman, SE (2005). Renovating the commons: Swedish health care reform in perspective. *Journal of Health Politics, Policy and Law*, 30(1–2):253–275.

Saltman RB, von Otter C (1987). Re-vitalizing public health care systems: a theory of public competition in Sweden. *Health Policy*, 7:21–40.

Saltman RB, von Otter C (1992a). *Planned markets and public competition: strategic reform in northern European health systems*. Buckingham, Open University Press.

Saltman RB, von Otter C (1992b). Reforming the Swedish health system in the 1990s: the emerging role of public firms. *Health Policy*, 21:143–154.

Saltman RB, von Otter C, eds. (1995). *Implementing planned markets: balancing social and economic responsibility*. Buckingham, Open University Press.

Saltman RB, Busse R, Mossialos E, eds. (2002). *Regulating entrepreneurial behaviour in European health care systems*. Buckingham, Open University Press.

Saltman RB, Figueras J, Busse R, eds. (2004). *Social health insurance systems in western Europe*. Maidenhead, Open University Press.

Scott WR et al. (2000). *Institutional change and healthcare organizations: from professional dominance to managed care*. Chicago, IL, University of Chicago Press.

Smith PC et al., eds. (2009). *Performance measurement for health system improvement: experiences, challenges and prospects*. Cambridge, Cambridge University Press.

Succi MJ, Alexander JA (1999). Physician involvement in management and governance: the moderating effects of staff structure and composition. *Health Care Management Review*, 24:33–44.

Tuohy CH (2003). Agency, contract and governance: shifting shapes of accountability in the health care arena. *Journal of Health Politics, Policy and Law*, 28(2–3):195–215.

Van Doorslaer E et al. (2000). Equity in the delivery of health care in Europe and the US. *Journal of Health Economics*, 19(5):553–583.

Wensing M et al. (2001). *Factors in theories on behaviour change to guide implementation and quality improvement in health care. Technical Report for the Rebeqi project*. Brussels, European Commission Fifth Framework, Directorate-General for Research (Contract no. QLRT-00657).

West MA, Anderson NR (1996). Innovation in top management teams. *Journal of Applied Psychology*, 81(6):680–693.

Zablocki E (2007). Best practices for public hospital governance. *Great Boards*, Fall:1–7.

Chapter 3
Mapping new governance models for public hospitals

Richard B. Saltman, Hans F.W. Dubois and Antonio Durán

3.1 Learning from country case studies

Chapters 1 and 2 reviewed in some detail the changing operating environment with which public hospitals are faced. This chapter explores the degree of change taking place in the way public hospitals (along with non-profit-making private institutions in the Netherlands) are governed in Europe. Using eight commissioned case studies and the conceptual framework previously established, the chapter looks closely at the development of new modalities of public hospital governance on the production side of the health system (Saltman, 1994). It examines in particular the degree to which governance arrangements have been affected by the ongoing redefinition of the boundaries of care, increased complexity in the relationship between stakeholders and the growing importance of new networks of power (for example, based on changing IT). Emphasis is placed on analysing the degree and content of decision-making autonomy at the meso-institutional level as the essential variable in hospital governance. Pursuing an initial review, the study examines key countries known for adopting new models of public hospital governance, and thus provides an initial mapping and assessment of the changes that have occurred to date. Ideally, some of the main structural and organizational lessons will be relevant for other publicly operated hospital systems elsewhere, both in Europe and beyond.

Seven of the eight countries have redesigned governance models with a greater degree of decision-making autonomy introduced into some or all of their publicly owned hospitals. The eighth country, the Netherlands, has hospitals that, while no longer publicly owned (all publicly owned hospitals were transformed to non-profit-making foundation ownership by 1991), are important to this study, being at the private end of the continuum in terms of independence and autonomy, and thereby establishing a reference point for evaluating how far these new public hospital models have developed from their directly administered public peers.

In terms of overall funding and system characteristics, the eight studied countries have four different types of funding arrangements. Norway, England, Portugal and Spain are predominantly tax-funded systems; Israel has a mixed tax/SHI model, and Estonia and the Czech Republic have implemented a new post-1990 central European hybrid form of state-controlled SHI funds. The Netherlands has a different hybrid SHI system, combining a state-mandated nominal premium paid by each individual with a central government-run pool that collects a fixed percentage of each employee's salary (subsequently reimbursed to the individual by employers, for those who work).

Taken together, observations drawn from these eight country cases enable some initial conclusions to be drawn regarding overall patterns of change and developments in public hospital governance across Europe. Responses in each of the case studies to eight key questions relating to the country's hospital governance structure are tabulated in the Appendix, presented after Chapter 4 at the end of Part I.

3.2 Applying the analytic framework categories

3.2.1 Institutional dimension

In most semi-autonomous models of hospital governance in Europe, the hospital management makes decisions regarding major *structural parameters*, such as the hospital's service configuration, number of beds and the degree of focus on outpatient services. For major resource-related questions, however, regional (Norway, Spain and England) or central governments typically maintain leverage to various degrees. For decisions relating to the level of clinical services offered (district/secondary/tertiary), there is additional input by insurers in models in which sick funds play an important role in health care financing (in the Czech Republic, and for sick fund-owned hospitals in Israel), however, with somewhat more autonomy for the hospitals.

In terms of *employment relations* within these semi-autonomous models, medical specialists are mostly salaried employees, with pay levels either controlled by national agreement (in government and sick fund-owned hospitals, and private non-profit-making hospitals in Israel) or, as in several of the models in Spain, salaries are subject to additional local negotiation at the hospital level. However, some semi-autonomous models do shift physicians to independent contractors, with differential pay negotiated separately for each specialist, as is the case in limited liability and joint-stock companies in the Czech Republic, in the private hospital owned by the sickness fund in Israel, and in private non-profit-making institutions in the Netherlands. Labour unions generally play a less important role in these semi-autonomous hospitals. While they remain relatively important in several western European countries (England, Norway, Portugal and Spain), they have less significance in Israel, and little effective authority in the two central European countries (Estonia and the Czech Republic) or in the Netherlands (see section 3.3 for a more detailed analysis).

3.2.2 Financing dimension

Generally, *investment capital* for large new equipment, renovations and new buildings comes from owner investments and/or national government contributions, hospital funds and/or bank loans. Grants by the EU (Estonia, Portugal) and by charities (government- and sickness fund-owned hospitals in Israel) may play significant roles. In models closer to the private end of the spectrum (e.g. private hospitals with sickness funds as major owners), shareholders provide funds as well. For *operating capital* (day-to-day expenses: staff payroll, supplies and overheads such as heat and light), funding sources are somewhat different. Here, hospital resources, activity-based state financing (Portugal, Norway, Foundations in Spain), and – when applicable – insurance companies (Czech Republic) play a more prominent role.

With regard to the decision process, *capital investments* are usually initiated by the Management Board, then approved by the hospital's Supervisory Board and sometimes by the national or regional government. In Portuguese PEEHs, national government approval is needed beyond a specified magnitude of the investment: 2% of the hospital's statutory capital. For decisions concerning operating costs, the board generally has a relatively prominent role throughout the whole process (see section 3.3 for a more detailed discussion).

There is considerable variation in the extent to which hospitals can retain their *financial surpluses*. In traditional public hospitals – as in public institutions and agencies generally – any operating surplus remaining at the end of the budget year must be returned to the funding department, a requirement which dampens financial incentives for innovative and/or entrepreneurial behaviour within the public sector. Among the eight case studies, four distinct groups can be identified. At one end of the spectrum are hospital models in which hospitals remain unable to retain financial surpluses, such as the Czech Republic's public contributory organizations, as well as Public Healthcare Companies (*Empresa Pública Sanitaria*) in Spain within which surpluses must be given back to the regional government's finance department. Next are models in which the possibility to retain surpluses is conditional upon the decision of the owner – for example, sickness funds (Israeli sickness fund-owned hospitals) or regional governments (joint-stock companies and limited liability companies in the Czech Republic). A third group of models consists of hospitals which can retain surpluses, subject to considerable restrictions. In Administrative Concession (*Concesión Administrativa*) hospitals in Spain, surpluses can be retained up to a fixed annual profit rate, capped at 7.5%. Additional earnings – after taxes – should be reimbursed to the regional health authority. England's Self-governing Trusts can retain surpluses but are expected to break even over a three-year period. The fourth group consists of hospital models in which the institutions can retain their surpluses – this includes Dutch (private, non-profit-making) hospitals, Norwegian Regional Health Enterprises and all Estonian semi-autonomous hospital models.

3.2.3 Accountability framework

A key element in the accountability framework is the *Supervisory Board*, which is sometimes called a Board of Governors (England) or a Board of Trustees. Most hospital models included in this study include such a board. These boards supervise the activities of the Management Board/Executive Board. In some Israeli and Portuguese models, there is no Supervisory Board. These hospitals are controlled by sickness funds (sickness fund-owned hospitals in Israel) or by the national government (all ministry-owned hospitals in Israel, and public hospitals in Portugal). In Israel, government- and sickness fund-owned hospitals also do not have a Management Board, but are managed by individual CEOs with considerable authority.

In most models, the Supervisory Board appoints the *Management Board* or (as in Estonian Foundations) its head, who then appoints the other members. In several models (Czech Republic, Norway, Spain) the regional or municipal government appoints board members. In England, there is an interesting split. For Foundation Trusts, there are five non-executives and a chair approved by the Board of Governors, as well as five executives appointed by the Executive Board. For Self-governing Trusts, five non-executives and a chair are appointed by an independent commission and the Trust, while five executives are appointed by the Executive Board, with some involvement of the national government in CEO appointments.

With regard to size of the board, some models impose a maximum number of members, either nationally/regionally (PEEHs in Portugal), or statutorily (Estonian models), while others leave the decision to the discretion of the Supervisory Board (private non-profit-making hospitals in the Netherlands). Within the cases examined, the size usually varies between five and six members (PEEHs in Portugal, Public Healthcare Companies in Spain, and public contributory organizations in the Czech Republic) to 10 or more (England, Norway).[8] Rules regarding composition exist, for example in PEEHs in Portugal, in which one of the board members should be a clinical director (required to be a physician) and another a nurse director (a nurse).

Direct citizen participation is largely absent among the models examined. Board meetings must be open only in the Norwegian model and in Self-governing Trusts in England. Citizen members of English Foundation Trusts can vote for representatives on the Board of Governors. Several models include ombudsmen and spokespersons, and/or publish minutes of board meetings. In the sickness fund-owned hospitals in Israel, sickness fund members and Labour Federation members have an indirect voice through their organizations.

3.2.4 Operational governance boundaries

Generally, in the semi-autonomous governance models discussed here, the hospital makes decisions independently, without formal operating boundaries set by government. However, for models in which politicians sit on the boards or where they can appoint board members, this may mean that there is still government involvement in decision-making. Furthermore, informal boundaries may exist (e.g. in Norway) that restrict hospital and/or management decisions. Estonian models have explicit boundaries without much room to depart from fixed objectives. In some cases, boundaries are enforced implicitly by financial dependence (Estonia, PEEHs in Portugal). In the Israeli models, operational governance boundaries are established by planning decisions and staffing-level requirements, both determined by the Ministry of Health. For the Israeli (private non-profit-making) sickness fund-owned hospitals, an additional element in setting boundaries includes the financial decisions of the sickness fund (owner).

---

8 Broadly speaking, they have between 6 and 12 members – the range indicated by corporate governance literature as being most effective (Denis, 2001, reprinted in Eeckloo et al., 2004), with a larger number hindering effective decision-making, lengthening the process and reducing the commitment of the individual members.

3.2.5 Internal operational governance

In all hospital models included in this study, the management of the hospital can make decisions affecting the hospital's internal professional structures, such as the numbers and functions of chiefs of service. The only exceptions are models with self-employed physicians working within the hospital, such as in the Dutch private non-profit-making hospitals. In all hospital models, these powers are constrained by public sector regulations. Furthermore, formal authority or "the right to decide" can deviate considerably from real authority or "the effective control over decisions" (Aghion & Tirole, 1997) in a hospital setting.

While none of the models have explicit caps on the cost of the organizational structures, or "transaction costs", in practice there are substantial cost concerns. In England, the NHS has been strongly encouraged by the new coalition government to reduce its management costs. In the hospital governance models examined, hospital management teams generally have the freedom to organize the hospital's own internal operational structures (architecture and routines – operational methodology, clearly mapped processes, benchmarks/best practice standards, etc.) and authority and responsibility relations ("departmentalization", staff, committees and groups, decentralization, coordination systems, number and organization of the middle management). This does not mean that all is decided by the hospital board alone. Department heads, for example, often have an important stake in the decision-making process. Regulatory standards for care delivery also play a role.

In most models, the hospitals can decide when to hire and fire employees. For micro-level, specific hiring and firing decisions and for relatively large hospitals, decisions may be made at the department level. In the case of autonomous groups of specialists working in the hospital (Netherlands), the hospital's management may have little effective influence.

3.2.6 Decision-making capacity versus responsibility, internal monitoring and incentive systems

In several of these cases, a discrepancy exists between the decision-making capacity of the hospital board and what it is responsible for overseeing. For example, in all publicly owned Israeli hospital models, the hospital management has little or no control over workforce costs, which amount to about 70% of total expenditure, yet it defines specific objectives for the hospital's overall mission, including providing safe, effective care, staying within budget, excellence in care, teaching and research. In the Norwegian model, similarly, objectives have been characterized as "too detailed".

Decisions relating to the inclusion of new drugs and treatments and the setting up of clinical trials are made by different combinations of hospital board, individual physicians and departments, and governments. Some models have separate commissions to deal with clinical trials (Estonia) or with the inclusion of new drugs (Spain).

In several of the models, performance-related incentives can affect staff income. In other models, hospitals cannot set such incentives. In Spanish Public Healthcare Foundations (*Fundaciones Públicas Sanitarias*) and in Norway, most employees are salaried, with no room for incentive-based payment. In other models, hospitals are entirely (English Foundation Trusts) or partly (English Self-governing Trusts) free to set such incentives. Often there are restrictions, as in Czech public contributory organizations, in which the basic salary level is set by governmental decree, but the hospital can allocate bonuses. In practice, though, the hospital system in Estonia has by far the largest share of income affected by incentivization (25%). In other models, incentive-based payment does not affect more than between 8% (Portuguese PEEHs, and Spanish *Consortia*) and 15% (Spanish Public Healthcare Companies). A larger proportion of salaries can be affected by such incentives in the case of private hospitals (two thirds in Estonia) or in terms of managers' salaries (35% in Spanish Public Healthcare Companies). Incentive systems are either defined by means of consensus of the organization as a whole (Portuguese PEEHs, Israeli private non-profit-making hospitals), or agreed with the individual staff members (Israeli government-owned hospitals).

With regard to performance indicators, different patterns can be observed. One group of models (Spanish Public Healthcare Company) requires hospitals to apply such indicators or, often, hospitals within certain models apply them voluntarily (Estonian joint-stock companies and foundations). These data are sometimes included in the hospitals' annual reports. Some of these models, in addition (Estonian joint-stock companies and foundations) or exclusively (Portuguese PEEHs), share performance data internally, through full-fledged internal benchmarking systems (Czech limited liability companies), intranet (Portuguese PEEHs) or – more informally – by email (some Estonian joint-stock companies and foundations). Lastly, there are also models in which these data remain unpublished and are not shared internally, such as the Israeli and English models.

Hospitals can decide on parameters for monitoring day-to-day activity. Often, there are minimum data requirements to be collected for the national or regional government, such as data relating to patient flows (all Israeli hospitals), or monthly reporting on waiting lists and three-monthly reporting on the financial situation (*Consortia* hospitals in Spain). In the models examined, the Management/Executive Board decides which criteria will be used to evaluate whether key objectives have been achieved, with an important role for the department heads, especially in the Netherlands and – in all but the private – Israeli models.

3.3 Key issues in the different hospital models

The models of meso-level hospital governance already described vary on a wide range of structural and organizational parameters. While they resemble each other in certain fundamental characteristics, these hospital models typically vary considerably in how the particular activities or bodies are constructed. This mix of clear commonalities combined with widely differentiated specificities indicates the complexities involved in drawing conclusions about the broad dimensions of these governance models, as well as their potential applicability to other hospitals and/or in other countries and health care systems.

Utilizing the structural characteristics presented earlier, as well as the more detailed descriptions of hospital activities and behaviour in the case studies themselves, this section explores more closely several key structural similarities and differences that define these models of hospital governance. In particular, this section emphasizes elements of meso-level decision-making that involve the hospital Supervisory Board, and its relations with other key actors, such as elected politicians and unions. This focus reflects the simple reality that the Supervisory Board sits at the heart of meso-level hospital governance, and exercises or superintends whatever degree of autonomy the hospital has in its decision-making activities.

3.3.1 Legal status

There is considerable variation in the formal designation and legal status of public hospitals in seven of the country case studies. Among the four northern and central European cases, as described in Chapter 2, these new semi-autonomous models of hospital governance range from "trusts" to "foundations", and "state enterprises" to "joint-stock companies". Among the two Iberian cases, there are six different models, each with differing degrees of formal (and actual) autonomy. In Israel, the four different legal definitions of hospital also generate differing degrees of formal authority, although in this case hospitals directly managed and owned by the Ministry of Health also have considerable decision-making autonomy for up to 30% of their annual budget.

The formal legal status in the other case study – the Netherlands – is relatively new (the last conversion from public to non-profit-making private foundation took place in 1991) and is seen to be not entirely stable. The case study notes that the Minister of Health, Welfare and Sport intervened directly when one hospital approached bankruptcy, despite its formally private status, out of stated concern for the patients' continuity of care. Further, the Dutch government has put forward legislation to once again change the legal basis of Dutch hospitals, this time to an "enterprise with a social dimension" (see Chapter 9).

In addition to differing levels of formal autonomy, the new models of public hospital governance also have considerable variation in who their "owners" are. Being publicly owned institutions, the hospital owners in seven of the eight countries (all except Netherlands) were typically national, regional or municipal governments, or – as in Estonia – a combination of national and municipal governments together. However, Dutch hospitals are private non-profit-making entities owned by a domestically chartered foundation. In the Israeli case, one private non-profit-making hospital is owned by a foreign foundation (Hadassah in New York) and another by a domestic non-profit-making enterprise (an Israeli sickness fund – now called "health funds").

The cases suggest, however, that the notion of private non-profit-making ownership of a hospital is often deceptive. Whereas this category of ownership may indicate true independence of operation in other sectors of the economy (social service, education), in the health sector, national governments in Europe often reserve the right to intervene as they believe appropriate. Hence, in the Netherlands, although hospitals are formally privately owned, the Minister of Health, Welfare and Sport nonetheless has the ability to intervene. In Israel, the private non-profit-making hospital still requires agreement from the Ministry of Health, Welfare and Sport for major capital- or service-related decisions.

3.3.2 Importance of the Supervisory Board

As already described, a central element in nearly all models is the establishment of a hospital-level body that is formally responsible for each hospital's activities and performance. In nearly all cases (exceptions being the few privatized hospitals in the Czech Republic, several new for-profit hospitals recently established in Estonia, and Israel, where ministry-owned hospitals have no board and non-profit-making private, sick fund-owned and profit-making hospitals have boards that are not appointed by politicians), appointment to these boards is carried out by political authorities, at either local municipal (Estonia), regional (Spain, Czech Republic) or national (Norway, England, Portugal) level. In the Netherlands, where hospitals are not publicly owned but are private non-profit-making entities, the Supervisory Board is self-renewing and appointments are made with no political input or review. In a different type of direct local politics, for the Foundation Trusts introduced after 2004 in England, the defined membership of the Trust (which includes both patients and hospital staff) vote for governors, who in turn appoint the head of the Supervisory Board.

As discussed, the size of the Supervisory Boards varies; however, there is a notable tendency to view smaller boards of between five and seven members as being more effective. Boards in Estonia vary in size, while Dutch boards – a useful example from the non-profit-making private sector – typically have six or seven members. Larger numbers are seen as a reflection of formal rather than actively engaged supervision.

In terms of the membership of the board, in several of these new models there are at least a few active politicians, typically placed on the board to speak for the interests of the political body they represent. The actual arrangements can vary; for example, in Andalusia, the Public Healthcare Company model has one board member who represents the Regional Ministry of Health and one representing the Regional Ministry of Finance, whereas in Estonia, the Supervisory Board of each hospital often has active politicians representing local government (although recently some politicians have been opting to appoint technical professionals onto hospital boards).

There are contradictory opinions regarding whether to appoint physicians from a hospital to its Supervisory Board (as opposed to its Management or Executive Board – see, for example, Molinari and colleagues (1995)). In Portugal, for the post-2005 PEEH hospitals, the chief physician of the hospital always sits on the Supervisory Board. However, in the non-profit-making hospitals of the Netherlands, no physicians are voted onto the Supervisory Board. This Dutch model reflects the view that "you can't supervise yourself" (see Maarse and Lodewick's contributions in Chapter 9).

3.3.3 Functions of Supervisory Boards

The central role of these Supervisory Boards can be described in several different ways. The stated formal role of these new boards has been to increase the scrutiny with which previously traditional public sector administration had approached the running and behaviour of these institutions. In England, the Foundation Trust boards were intended "to challenge managers, and to prevent groupthink" (Edwards, 2010; see also Chapter 8). In Estonia, the role of the Supervisory Board was seen as "to protect the public interest". However, it was also noted that, in practice, it was often the case that "managers trained their boards" (Edwards, 2010). In the non-profit-making private hospitals of the Netherlands, the role of the Supervisory Boards was strategic in focus: to review budgets, appoint accountants, approve mergers and appoint the Executive Board (e.g. hospital managers). Indeed, the role of the Supervisory Board was seen as more hortatory than exercising direct power: "arbitor, inspirator, diplomat". In the last analysis, however, in these Dutch private hospitals, "the Executive Board has final responsibility" (see Chapter 9).

Beyond the formal role of the Supervisory Boards, their practical responsibility has been surveillance specifically of the fiscal activities of the publicly owned but semi-autonomously operated hospitals to which they are appointed. The boards in nearly all of the eight country case studies focus first and foremost on budget, investment and working capital decisions. In this sense the boards typically are responsible for approving the strategic and operating proposals put forward by the hospital's Executive Board, and/or the hospital CEO. This is true of the Supervisory Boards of the Foundation Trusts in England, those of the Public Healthcare Company hospitals in Andalusia, the PEEH hospitals in Portugal, the state enterprise hospitals in Norway and the independently constituted public hospitals in Estonia. This emphasis on financial issues at both strategic and operating levels reflects the fundamental objective of these new public hospital models, in terms of improving the overall efficiency with which they deliver health services. Thus, while other issues – such as quality of care, patient safety, responsiveness to and satisfaction of patients – all play a role in the deliberations of these Supervisory Boards, it is their core concern with financial performance that has guided their activities to date.

An impending and as yet unresolved issue for Supervisory Boards in a number of the case study countries is the need to monitor and evaluate clinical performance and – more important than just process – to assess the medical efficacy of the actual clinical outcomes. This newly evolving concern is likely to generate a variety of additional board activities, integrating the boards more firmly into the day-to-day medical activities of the clinical staff – an area that thus far the Supervisory Boards have left to the discretion and more in-depth knowledge of the hospital managers (e.g. the CEOs and the Executive Boards). How this new set of outcome-based responsibilities will alter the relationship between the Supervisory Board and the rest of the hospital remains to be seen. It should be noted, of course, that this same concern with clinical performance and clinical outcomes is increasing across the whole of the European hospital sector (Smith et al., 2009), and thus will eventually influence the activities not just of the new governance models discussed here, but also of traditionally managed public hospitals and both non-profit-making and profit-making private institutions.

3.3.4 Frequency of Supervisory Board meetings

Although the Supervisory Board makes the final decision on most financial activities, as well as approving a variety of other matters proposed by the management team, the board itself has little ability to supervise day-to-day activities. In the best of circumstances, the board meets on a monthly basis, with the exceptions of Christmas and over the summer – which, for example in the Netherlands, means about eight times a year. In the Public Healthcare Company hospitals of Andalusia, the Supervisory Board meets twice a year. However, there can also be informal contact between the chairman of the Supervisory Board and the hospital management team. In one Dutch hospital, for example, the chair of the Supervisory Board met bi-weekly with the hospital CEO, and there was also frequent telephone and email contact between them (see Chapter 9). Further, in Estonia, for the several (new) profit-making private hospitals there, there was only one Board, combining supervisory and management responsibilities, which met several times weekly. Thus, it would appear reasonable to conclude that, in most instances, the Supervisory Boards in these new models of hospital governance across Europe exercised a rather distant, generally supportive – rather than actively involved – role in actual hospital decisions and behaviour.

3.3.5 Political influence on hospital decisions

A major objective of the new models was to create distance for both day-to-day and also some strategic decisions from the influence of political concerns and political actors. This distance was seen as essential to enable publicly owned hospitals to operate more efficiently and to make better use of their resources and capacities. However, these remain publicly owned hospitals, dependent upon (except to some extent Foundation Hospitals in England) publicly supplied capital, and accountable to the public sector for meeting overall financial and clinical standards. Thus, it is essential at the end of the day that these public institutions are held directly accountable for their outputs by their political directors. If public institutions are deemed necessary in order to maintain universal access to health, along with social cohesion, then an important evaluative role exists for society's political bodies in terms of these semi-autonomous public hospitals. That said, the question then arises regarding where to draw the boundary, how to find the correct balance between autonomy of decision-making and political accountability for these costly but essential publicly funded institutions.

The available evidence from the eight health system case studies suggests that, as hard as it is to define the appropriate balance between autonomy and political accountability, it is even harder to maintain that agreed balance once it is introduced. There appears to be an innate (if not natural) inclination on the part of political actors to seek to reassert greater control over these institutions, as well as for initial levels of autonomy of hospital decision-making to slip back towards greater direct political control over time. While the recent difficult economic situation has provided a convenient justification for this rollback of quasi-autonomous authority for these hospitals, clearly the impetus to restore more direct political authority runs deeper. In Portugal, for example, after the new public enterprise model was set up in 2005, there was a notable increase in political demands: "old habits began again in hospitals" (Raposo, 2010). In Andalusia in 2008, Public Healthcare Company hospitals were no longer allowed to retain any operating surplus internally, instead being required – as are traditionally managed public hospitals – to return this surplus to the Regional Ministry of Health at the end of the budget year. In Valencia, in the broadly autonomous *Consortia* model, the new CEO for the hospital is the former representative of the Regional Ministry of Health, who previously had been stationed in an office next door to the prior CEO in order to monitor his decisions. In England, a key reason for establishing the Foundation Trust model was to reassert the principle of quasi-independent decision-making for public hospitals after the prior model of Self-governing Trusts had seen its autonomous decision-making influence slowly eroded to much less than had originally been intended (Edwards, 2010).

One important explanation for the increased role of political actors reflects the central fact that, although these hospitals are semi-autonomous in their decision-making, they are also (in most cases, except in the Netherlands) publicly owned hospitals, spending (also in the Netherlands) one or another form of public funds, and thus there is considerable public concern that funds should be spent in a manner consistent with broader political and social objectives. For example, the Norwegian case study remarks that any effort to close a rural satellite hospital centre (Roros) will be blocked by the Ministry of Health (see Chapter 10). Elsewhere in the same case study, it is noted that "in some cases the Minister will have views and will directly influence Regional Boards" (see section 10.2). In the Netherlands, regarding formally independent hospitals chartered in the private non-profit-making sector, although "the national government wants to give back health care to society, always there are new regulations that signify greater interference. Politics is penetrating the hospital more and more. The hospitals are seen as part of the public sector, and thus under the direct control of the Ministry of Health" (Maarse, 2010). One stated justification for this tightening of political control is that "the Minister is responsible for service coverage, thus he'd have to approve a closing" (Maarse, 2010). Recently the Dutch Ministry of Health, Welfare and Sport has intervened in disputes regarding the size of hospital CEO salaries, on the basis that these are paid using public funds (Maarse, 2010).

Conversely, a major advantage of the state having ultimate political authority is that hospitals are not allowed to go bankrupt, abruptly leaving patients without a locally appropriate care provider. Even in the Dutch example, where hospitals are private institutions with no formal relationship to the Ministry of Health, Welfare and Sport, there was (as noted earlier) recently an instance whereby a hospital turned to the Ministry to stave off impending bankruptcy. The response of the Minister was instructive: the funds were provided, but the cost to the hospital was that the Minister then appointed his own representative to that formally private hospital's Supervisory Board, with veto power over major decisions (see Chapter 9).

Clearly for this type of political authority to be exerted in the Dutch health care system, in which the hospitals are all formally independent of the Ministry of Health, Welfare and Sport, suggests the extent of the political capacity for government to intervene. In the United Kingdom, it is well known among civil servants that in the case of a politically embarrassing situation and/or one that is threatening to patients, even if the hospital has been guaranteed independence of decision-making, the Minister of Health will inevitably seek to intervene. "Ministers invent ways to intervene, telling civil servants to 'find a way' to make it possible" (Edwards, 2010). While such intervention may be directed (as in Norway) towards protecting the public interest, it highlights the fragility of autonomous decision-making for publicly owned hospitals in all eight countries, regardless of formal ownership structure. In essence, the hospitals' grant of quasi-autonomy lasts only until they make a decision that does not align with the preferences of the sitting government. Depending on one's view, that short leash may be either a good or a bad thing; however, its existence does define the outer limit of institutional-level governance in these new public hospital models.

3.3.6 Union influence on hospital decisions

The role of unions regarding independent decision-making by public hospitals in these new governance models appears to vary across the eight countries studied. Classically, a key objective for introducing these new models has been to reduce the influence of lock-step union restrictions against the introduction of both flexible deployment of staff and flexible financial incentives tied to performance. In public hospitals, as elsewhere in the public sector, employee unions traditionally have sought to exercise their industrial and electoral power to support political actors who will maximize the benefit not to the organization but rather to its employees. This approach has often prevented public hospital management from taking advantage of new managerial mechanisms and potential efficiencies and savings in the operation of their institutions, resulting in greater expenditure of public funds along with longer waiting lists. Depending on the issue, labour union disputes over the introduction of new labour-saving technologies and/or equipment have also resulted in delayed improvements in quality of patient care. In addition, there have been long-running disputes regarding contracting out hotel and catering-related services, as well as laboratory testing.

In Spain, dealing with union issues is a very sensitive matter, especially for socialist-led governments at national and/or regional level. The strong role of the unions reflects their role in the development of post-Francoist Spain, along with their links to the often-dominant Socialist Party, both in Madrid and within many regional governments. One solution has been (as seen in Andalusia) to determine that all newly built hospitals from the mid-1990s would be structured as "public institutions under private law". By taking this approach, the new hospital's managers and Supervisory Board would resemble private sector businesses, having more flexibility in (among other areas) their negotiations with hospital sector labour unions. This approach resulted in a somewhat more fluid picture managerially, particularly with regard to granting financial incentives tied to performance to staff who meet or exceed their productivity targets. In Public Healthcare Company hospitals, the management can designate substantial funds for financial incentives at the clinic level. Administrative staff can receive up to 40% of their salary in incentive pay. For clinical staff, the picture is more complicated: if a clinic earns an incentive payment, the key individual (usually a physician) can receive 40% of those funds, while the other 60% must be distributed equally to all other members of the clinic staff, regardless of their input into the higher productive activities. This distribution is mandated by the labour unions, which are informed about all negotiations with clinical department chiefs, and which seek to balance any individual incentives with traditional union concerns regarding pay equality for non-rewarded staff.

In Norway, although all publicly owned hospitals have been transformed into the state enterprise model, decisions regarding financial incentives for individual physicians and staff members nonetheless remain difficult. As the Norwegian case study notes, "a more individual approach to wage setting would not be accepted by the unions" (see section 10.3).

Conversely, in Estonia's new hospital model, the role of unions is minimal in terms of managerial strategy and financial incentives for staff. Reflecting Estonia's extraordinary political shift since the early 1990s, from being a Soviet Republic, with hospital decision-making often being centralized to Moscow, to its current status as a Member State of the EU, as well as the dramatic change in economic status that has accompanied this political shift, there is little sympathy in Estonia for strong union intervention in hospital efficiency matters. Reflecting this major contextual shift, unions in Estonia are quite weak, with their influence confined to wage-related matters, and for these often only the ability to take their complaints to the Ministry of Social Affairs in hopes of obtaining a political fix. The unions in Estonia appear to have only a marginal role in the setting and implementation of financial incentives and other managerial initiatives at the individual hospital level.

In the Netherlands, which again as a system of private non-profit-making hospitals – can serve as the outer benchmark for what might be possible in terms of meso-level governance models for publicly owned hospitals, the past history of strong union influence over national political decision-making no longer applies in the current economic context. At the hospital level, unions have little formal leverage over decisions made either by the management (executive) or the Supervisory Boards. Given Dutch culture and social traditions, the medical staff still have a powerful role in how Dutch hospitals develop, and in the introduction of new managerial mechanisms such as financial incentive payments. Indeed, the medical staff play a major role in the development of the hospital budget, and, if they decide to collectively complain about the management to the Supervisory Board, stand a good chance of being able to have senior management dismissed. However, the formal role of unions in these activities is not strong.

3.3.7 Supervisory Board relations with hospital management

A key governance question relates to the ability of the Supervisory Board to steer the hospital's management team, for example its CEO and, in most of the case study countries, its Executive Board. Traditionally, the Executive Board – based on its intimate knowledge of operating behaviour – formulates proposals that it then presents to the Supervisory Board for approval. The role of the Supervisory Board is to provide guidance, support and ultimately make a decision; however, the impetus for new activity comes from the managerial team. Thus, the Supervisory Board's role is one of being "coach, arbitor, inspirator, diplomat" (Maarse, 2010), concentrating on budget, finance, new investment, and capital issues. While this description reflects the actual situation in the Netherlands, with its independent private institutions, it also reflects the type of interactions often seen at any hospital for which there is an external Supervisory Board. It reflects the reality that the Supervisory Board is not in a position to run the hospital itself, and thus must work with and through the hospital's senior managers.

The second, trickier role for the Supervisory Board arises when the hospital's medical staff sidestep the Executive Board in order to petition the Supervisory Board for help and support with a specific problem or issue. Typically this occurs when there has been a serious split between the hospital's senior management and the leading physicians, and the intention of the physicians is to try to have the CEO and/or other senior managers dismissed. While in theory the Supervisory Board can try to patch the relationships back together, it is not uncommon for a board to decide that the CEO – evidently being unable to make common cause with her/his physicians – has become a liability in terms of the good functioning of the hospital. Since it is difficult to replace all the hospital physicians, the typical solution to this situation is for the hospital to hire a new CEO.

3.3.8 Ability of new models to improve performance/outcomes

Semi-autonomous hospital models are seen as being reasonably successful in most if not all of the eight countries studied in this volume. Despite the various difficulties detailed earlier, most of these hospitals have considerably more discretion in their operating decisions than their traditionally managed public peers, and at least some have a certain level of input in decisions regarding more strategic issues, such as budget, finance and capital development.

While not all these reconfigured hospitals are innovative in everything they do, many of them are more innovative than their directly managed public sector counterparts in such areas as financial incentives, hiring and firing, and patient responsiveness and satisfaction. Some of these hospitals have the important ability to retain their budget surplus for use in the next budget year, and many of them in Andalusia, as well as among the Foundation Trusts in England, no longer run annual deficits. In Portugal, a study of the first wave (2002–2005) of more autonomous public hospitals found that there was "improvement in some areas: more efficiency of operation but with no loss of access or equity" (Raposo, 2010).

A further measure of the overall usefulness of these models is that they are popular with patients, and at the same time there is no concerted move by political actors to abolish these new models. On the contrary, in Andalusia, the political actors see the new models as opportunities to pilot managerial and clinical techniques that could in the future be applied to all public hospitals. In Spain there is a strong sense that the new models "are here to stay" (Alvarez, 2010).

In Norway, there is both a sense that the new models have improved the overall situation, and a concern that additional changes may be required in order to achieve the necessary performance and outcome levels. The relevant case study notes that, once the studied teaching hospital's CEO and head of the Supervisory Board were changed, the hospital was able within two years to transform a 10% deficit into a balanced budget. However, there is no certainty that the current overall model of state enterprise hospitals funded by the national government through regional boards is the final word on health system structure. On the contrary: there is a sense currently in Norway that additional centralization of control may be necessary to deal with the still unsustainable costs of the current system (Larssen, 2009;[9] Magnussen, Vrangbaek & Saltman, 2009).

In certain countries, such as the Netherlands and England, governments are directing the development of a hospital governance model under which medical specialists would be integrated into the management and governance structures. The effect of this policy has been limited due to a counter-strategy from organized medical specialists, led by self-employed physicians, in order to remain largely autonomous (Scholten & van der Grinten, 2002), but general hospitals are indeed increasingly held accountable as a whole by the public at large (Schaaf, 2000).

A further aspect of this political quandary concerns the extent to which the official rules governing the particular distribution of responsibilities can be abruptly altered in the case of perceived or real political necessity. Recently in the Netherlands, for example, when a private non-profit-making hospital teetered on bankruptcy, the Ministry of Health, Welfare and Sport intervened to provide the necessary funds, but then followed this by breaking all semblance of separation between the hospital's private non-profit-making status and the public sector, by placing a ministry representative on the hospital's Supervisory Board with veto power over all decisions (Maarse, 2010). In another recent example, public consternation at high salaries for hospital CEOs led the Netherlands' Ministry of Health, Welfare and Sport to intervene with "voluntary" restrictions which – if not adhered to – would then become mandatory salary regulations. Somewhat similarly, in the Public Healthcare Company model that has been developed since the mid-1990s for new hospitals in Andalusia in Spain, the Supervisory Board for each hospital includes a representative of both the Regional Ministry of Health and the Regional Ministry of Finance, each of which has veto power over board decisions (Alvarez, 2010; Huertas, 2010). Thus, in both the Dutch and Spanish cases, in quite different political systems with different models of health care financing and management, the final line under hospital decision-making was in fact drawn by the responsible political bodies, not the hospital itself. Additional instances can be cited in Estonia (municipal officials), in Portugal and in examples such as the 2009 Staffordshire Hospital incident in England (see Chapter 6). In reality, the practical balance between hospital autonomy and political control ultimately remains indistinct in these models, and the fundamental nature of the actual reforms thus requires continued assessment and evaluation.

---

9   Statement by B.-J. Larssen in joint Norwegian Ministry of Health/European Observatory on Health Systems and Policies seminar. Oslo, 26 October 2009.

As these examples relating to political balance suggest, the extent to which the existing balance between independent decision-making and political control can be characterized as either "good" or "bad" – in terms of the ability of the hospital sector to meet its obligations – is not easy to define. The answer lies obscured beneath the weight of academic evidence and experience, the expectations of the patient populations in the affected countries, the nature of the new models that have been introduced and, of course, the expectations, behaviour and fiscal situations within the municipal, regional or national governments concerned. How best to achieve a reasonable balance between institutional autonomy and political influence will likely continue to remain an unresolved but critical question.

3.4 References

Aghion P, Tirole J (1997). Formal and real authority in organizations. *Journal of Political Economy*, 105(1):1–29.

Alvarez A (2010). Author's workshop, 14 January. Granada, Andalusian School of Public Health.

Denis DK (2001). Twenty-five years of corporate governance research...and counting. *Review of Financial Economics*, 10(3):191–212.

Edwards N (2010). Author's workshop, 14 January. Granada, Andalusian School of Public Health.

Eeckloo K et al. (2004). From corporate governance to hospital governance. Authority, transparency and accountability of Belgian non-profit hospitals' board and management. *Health Policy*, 68:1–15.

Huertas M (2010). Author's workshop, 14 January. Granada, Andalusian School of Public Health.

Maarse H (2010). Author's workshop, 14 January. Granada, Andalusian School of Public Health.

Magnussen J, Vrangbaek K, Saltman RB, eds. (2009). *Nordic health care systems: recent reforms and current policy challenges*. Maidenhead, Open University Press.

Molinari C et al. (1995). Does the hospital board need a doctor? The influence of physician board participation on hospital financial performance. *Medical Care*, 33(2):170–185.

Raposo V (2010). Author's workshop, 14 January. Granada, Andalusian School of Public Health.

Saltman RB (1994). A conceptual overview of recent health care reforms. *European Journal of Public Health*, 4:287–293.

Schaaf JH (2000). *Hoe een ziekenhuis effectief te besturen? [How to govern effectively a hospital?]* [Doctoral dissertation]. Brabant, Catholic University Brabant.

Scholten GRM, van der Grinten TED (2002). Integrating medical specialists and hospitals; the growing relevance of collective organisation of medical specialists for Dutch hospital governance. *Health Policy*, 62:131–139.

Smith PC et al., eds. (2009). *Performance measurement for health system improvement: experiences, challenges and prospects.* Cambridge, Cambridge University Press.

Chapter 4
Conclusions and remaining issues

Richard B. Saltman and Antonio Durán

The concept of "hospital governance" represents a relatively new, more broadly based approach to hospital-related policy and to health policy analysis. Its emergence since the early 2000s reflects the growing number of political, financial and technical as well as social and professional factors that affect hospital sector decision-making, and that both policy-makers and hospital directors increasingly have to address.

This search for a new approach that is simultaneously cohesive and comprehensive has incorporated elements from predecessors such as New Public Management, as well as more than 25 years of experience developing governance concepts in the private corporate world (Jessop, 1995). In the health sector, however, these more general concepts have had to be modified to reflect the complexity of incorporating both macro national/political and meso institutional-level decision-making for the predominantly publicly owned hospitals in many European countries. National policy-makers in these countries have focused particularly on the usefulness of adopting private sector governance principles and strategies to improve the quality and efficiency of their public services, an interest which also has extended to education, elderly care and other social service areas, as well as the health sector.

4.1 Observations on public hospital autonomy

Within the health sector, these broad policy intentions have led quite quickly to the complex issue of institutional autonomy, and the boundaries within which publicly owned, publicly accountable organizations – especially hospitals – ought to be able to chart their own course. As mentioned in the Introduction, institutional autonomy is believed by some researchers to be a key factor in improving outcomes that policy-makers seek to achieve: quality of care, clinical outcomes and patient responsiveness (Bloom et al., 2010). This suggests that institutional autonomy is a central factor in determining the degree of success of recent public hospital governance reforms.

As considered in considerable detail in Chapter 3, the issue of decision-making autonomy for hospitals is complex and multifaceted. Not only do operating (or micro-level management) and capital issues come into play, but also numerous other factors that compose the concept of "governance": social responsibility, public accountability and good stewardship, as well as the more nuts-and-bolts issues of staff employment, professional responsibility, union authority and a range of practical political and financial decisions that are part of running institutions with budgets of hundreds of millions of euros, pounds, crowns or shekels.

The result is that, for all practical purposes, no publicly owned hospital is, or can ever expect to be, fully autonomous. The real-world issue for different strategies of meso-level hospital governance necessarily becomes the degree of autonomy, and over which factors of institutional life. The most that public hospitals can aspire to is to be "semi-autonomous", to have a limited degree of institutional independence within clearly defined but rigorously enforced decision-making boundaries. Moreover, that degree of autonomy may not be legally guaranteed, and frequently can be changed with little notice, should newly elected politicians prefer – or a change in the political environment suggest the usefulness of – tighter restrictions on hospital-based decision-making. In practice, then, some 20 years after these reforms began, a major operational issue for hospital governance still remains how well national policy-makers and hospital leaders can define the organizational dimensions and boundaries of the new "public firms" and "quasi-markets" that were first introduced in the early 1990s.

The descriptive materials presented in Chapter 3 indicate three different types of hospital governance reform introduced among the eight case study countries. The central variable, in keeping with the above discussion, is the degree of overall decision-making autonomy at institutional level, and the key factors that affect that outcome. As depicted in Table 4.1, the three different governance reforms can be termed "maximal semi-autonomy", "considerable semi-autonomy" and "restricted semi-autonomy".

Table 4.1 *Three types of public hospital governance reforms*

	Degree of political commitment	Degree of union resistance	Degree of structural change	Staff/ employee status
Restricted semi-autonomy	Weaker	Stronger	Minor	Salaried
Considerable semi-autonomy	Mixed	Weaker	Substantial	Salaried/incentives
Maximal semi-autonomy	Stronger	Not a factor	Systemic	Term-limited contracts

This three-part typology regarding degree of autonomy, in turn, can be used to construct a continuum of the degrees of semi-autonomy that hospitals (public as well as the non-profit-making private hospitals in the Netherlands and Israel) actually have in practice in each of the eight case study countries. Table 4.2 highlights the degree to which each type relates to traditional command-and-control notions of direct political authority, at one end of the conceptual spectrum, and full private profit-making autonomy, at the other.

Table 4.2 *Continuum of hospital governance strategies*

Command and control	Restricted semi-autonomy	Considerable semi-autonomy	Maximal semi-autonomy	Fully independent private
	Norway ↔			
	Portugal ⟵⟶			
	Israel ⟵————⟶			
	Estonia ⟵—⟶			
	Czech Republic ⟵——⟶			
		England ⟵⟶		
	Spain ⟵————————⟶			
			Netherlands ⟵⟶	

Several caveats are necessary at this point. First, full private sector-style autonomy is itself limited, still restrained by broad macro-level national policies, expectations and regulations. Profit-making private hospitals, like all non-profit-making private and publicly operated hospitals, must follow a substantial number of clinical, environmental, labour-related, financial and also political policies, as established by national political legislatures and executives (Saltman & Busse, 2002). However, private institutions typically do have considerable (although not absolute) decision-making autonomy with regard to operational issues, such as hiring/firing staff, initiating/closing services and a wide range of capital, operating, financing and budget issues. Thus, even fully private hospitals are subject to some macro-level political constraints at the meso-institutional level of hospital governance.

A second caveat concerns non-profit-making private hospitals, at least in Europe (their legal status is different in the United States, see Weisbrod, 1988). As Maarse and Lodevick note at several points in Chapter 9 (regarding hospitals in the Netherlands), the private non-profit-making category of hospitals is neither permanent nor particularly stable. Previously, all publicly owned hospitals were required to shift to the current category and at present the Dutch Government is considering requiring all hospitals to shift their legal status again – this time to a newly created category termed an "enterprise with a social purpose". Thus, much like the degree of semi-autonomy for public hospitals, the non-profit-making status of Dutch hospitals is somewhat arbitrary and may be changed at the discretion of the sitting national government. The key observation here is that the legal designation of a hospital does not represent a permanent category of law, and thus their non-profit-making private status continues only so long as the relevant national and/or regional/municipal government remains in agreement. As implied in Bevan's comment cited in the Introduction, this agreement could well be rescinded under fiscal or performance-related pressure.

With these caveats in mind, the distribution presented in Table 4.2 highlights a number of interesting relationships. Under the "restricted autonomy" category, one finds Norway, where the Ministry of Health and Care Services retains the right to veto hospital-level decisions regarding closures/capital issues, as well as several of Spain's five new models, in particular the Public Healthcare Company, in which the hospital Board of Supervisors includes a representative of the regional government's Ministry of Health and of its Ministry of Finance, each with veto power. Spain's *Consortia* model, however, falls under the middle category of "considerable autonomy," where it is joined in part by Portugal's PEEH model and, to a degree, the public hospitals in Israel (even though they are owned by the Ministry of Health) and also the private non-profit-making hospitals in Israel (which still must satisfy ministry concerns for larger operating and capital decisions). Other models that fit under this intermediate category are Self-governing Trusts in England, as well as foundations in Estonia and semi-budgetary organizations in the Czech Republic. Models that have "maximal autonomy" include the limited-stock companies in Estonia and the Czech Republic, as well as Foundation Trusts in England. Lastly, and reflective of the earlier discussion regarding the legal status of private non-profit-making organizations, the "maximal autonomy" category also includes private non-profit-making hospitals in the Netherlands.

Several intriguing implications for future policy can be drawn from Table 4.2. A key point is that the range of options displayed in the table reinforces the perception that different countries have approached public hospital governance reform in different ways, and in particular by granting considerably different degrees of meso-level institutional autonomy. One important question will be the extent of cross-learning among countries, with national policy-makers in one country being influenced by the degree of semi-autonomous decision-making granted to public hospitals in another country's model. Some would argue that this has already happened, pointing to the genesis of England's Foundation Trusts in Spain's Foundation model, and to Norway's state enterprises as having been influenced by England's first-round model of Self-governing Trusts.

A second intriguing question is whether the mix in Europe of different models of semi-autonomous decision-making is changing: specifically, whether it is moving either towards the "restricted autonomy" model – as some evidence from Spain, Norway and Portugal suggests that political actors are reasserting more authority – or whether the general trend is towards the "maximal autonomy" model, as some recent activity in Estonia – and, to a lesser degree, the replacement in England of Self-governing Trusts with Foundation Trusts, along with other efforts to expand hospital autonomy – might suggest.

Overall, it would appear that opinions are still divided, with no dominant trend apparent among the eight country cases. Additional study of decision-making autonomy for public hospitals in other countries in which change is occurring in their governance models – for instance, France and Poland have recently introduced reforms – may prove helpful in this respect. Moreover, policy-makers will likely require quantitative evidence from the micro-managerial level – for example, relating to hospital performance and outcomes data – before making further changes to their governance models.

The value of such quantitative assessments is hinted at in the initial conclusion by Bloom and colleagues (2010) that greater decision-making autonomy in combination with other institutional characteristics (large size, professional management, a highly competitive operating environment) may generate better clinical outcomes. This possibility can only serve to strengthen the attractiveness to national health policy-makers of semi-autonomous public models generally. Moreover, this evidence regarding better clinical performance in public hospitals needs to be balanced against the outcome of research into the relative clinical performance of profit-making compared with non-profit-making hospitals. Contrary to some analysts' assumptions favouring private profit-making hospitals (e.g. Harding & Preker, 2003), the preponderance of comparative studies appears to demonstrate that profit-making hospitals are not more clinically effective than their non-profit-making private counterparts (Jeurissen, 2010; Vaillencourt-Rosenau, 2003). From a policy-maker's perspective, then, it would appear that further development of semi-autonomous public models – given their close resemblance in operating behaviour to private non-profit-making institutions – may serve as a suitable policy response in some countries to the emerging (or potential) challenge of profit-making hospitals.

Thus far, this discussion of hospital autonomy has been broadly conceptual in nature. Practically speaking, however, policy-makers seeking to implement a more rational and/or effective governance regime also face concrete country-specific circumstances that should be considered. These can be illustrated by the practical characteristics of existing patterns of hospital governance in one case study country – Israel – where, officially, the public hospitals are owned and directly operated by the Ministry of Health, but where, in practical terms, a variety of different levels of operating autonomy exist, both formally and informally.

As the Israeli case indicates, in practice the CEOs of public hospitals have substantial decision-making autonomy under the general political umbrella of official ministry control. Moreover, as part of the modus vivendi that has been worked out, elements of this de facto autonomy have been legitimized by the establishment of "health corporations" under specific authorizing legislation, allowing hospitals to engage in a wide range of additional entrepreneurial activities and to retain the revenue generated by those activities.

A number of policy implications flow from this pragmatic policy strategy. First, although formally managed and controlled by the Ministry of Health, in reality Israeli public hospitals already have substantial operating autonomy in terms of certain activities – to a greater or lesser extent, depending on the hospital. In addition to the health corporations, for example, hospitals can also seek philanthropic contributions for capital investment, which are rarely overruled by the Ministry of Health.

Second, since public hospitals already have a considerable degree of operating autonomy, any effort by the Ministry of Health to formally restructure hospital governance arrangements towards a "public firm" or other more autonomous arrangement might well, in real terms (if actually enforced) represent a reduction rather than an enhancement of effective operating autonomy. This is of particular concern given the likelihood – as argued earlier – that the hospital of the next 20 years will differ considerably from the institutions of the past, hence the policy importance of developing new models of governance that do not reduce the ability of these institutions to respond appropriately to their rapidly changing environment.

Third, in turn, official decisions relating to designing new governance models will need to fit the new structure to the existing functions that have already been developed through independent decision-making in the Israeli public hospitals' day-to-day operations. Otherwise, the new, formally more autonomous model may again represent a reduction in real institutional autonomy and/or require that existing activities be curtailed.

Fourth, it is hardly surprising to find that hospitals led by physicians – as is the case in all Israeli public hospitals – would seek to expand the hospital's zone of decision-making independence. Considerable research about physician behaviour in several countries documents the consistent efforts of hospital specialists to carve out areas of operational freedom as heads of clinics or other clinical units (Young & Saltman, 1985; Saltman, 1985; Saltman & de Roo, 1989). Thus, qualified doctors as CEOs can be expected to continue the autonomy-seeking behaviour they demonstrated earlier in their professional lives. This observation, in turn, suggests that CEOs of public hospitals who are doctors can be expected to seek out informal opportunities for autonomous decision-making, in ways that indicate the Israeli experience may not be unique to that one health care system.

These practical observations all serve to reinforce the degree to which, practically speaking, the process of defining, regulating and steering autonomy in public hospitals operates in is part of a shifting terrain of complex, sometimes contradictory and/or counter-intuitive incentives that can create a treacherous environment for the design and implementation of effective governance reforms.

4.2 Further observations on public hospital governance

While this study focuses predominantly on the capacity for independent decision-making at the meso-institutional level, a number of other important institutional-level issues have also been raised. The case study review in Chapter 3 explored the role of the Executive or Management Board, the relationship between the Management Board and the Supervisory Board, the relationship between the hospital staff – particularly the physicians – with both the Management and Supervisory Boards, the role of financial incentives in shifting clinically related behaviour of physicians and other professional staff, and the relationship between public sector unions (where they play a role) and both boards. All of these roles and relationships form part of the meso-level governance framework, and the evidence from the case studies can provide a useful perspective on each of them.

4.2.1 Institutional accountability

While the case study evidence can be contradictory and is necessarily context specific, there is overall consensus that accountability is a desirable element in democratic societies; that each society has to find its own model to confront its challenges (as opposed to copying others, while still learning from each other's experiences); that this should be done in ways that are harmonious with the rest of the institutional map of the country; that clear roles and responsibilities facilitate effective operations; and that good operational decision-making (the real day-to-day responsibilities and limitations of what goes on at the hospital director level) helps service delivery institutions to achieve their objectives.

4.2.2 Staff involvement

Hospital staff involvement in the decision-making process seems desirable for making well-informed governance decisions and for ensuring a smooth implementation process. Conflicting interests, strategic voting, and occasional mutual distrust will arise, however, and mechanisms to ensure effective decision-making will be important. Effective governance thus includes ensuring that Supervisory and Management Boards are strong as well as that they apply meaningful consultation processes with physicians, staff and other stakeholders.

4.2.3 Public involvement

As public funds are centrally involved in financing health care in democratic European societies, accountability to the public is increasingly paramount. As a consequence, community representation in institution-level governance needs to be more than a facade. However, transparency should be implemented in a way that limits the risk of boards being stifled and decision-making slowed down. Chapter 3 noted some advantages of increased citizen participation and ways that this can take form, each with its own risks. Regular but not "too" regular, open, and well-publicized consultation meetings and frequently but not "too" frequently rotating community representation on supervisory boards may be desirable.

4.2.4 Size of boards

There appears to be little clear-cut evidence regarding the best size for Supervisory and Management Boards. While Supervisory Boards should not be too large, in some countries they seem effective with as few as six or seven members (the Netherlands and Estonia). Management Boards may have three or four members (typically including a managing physician and a finance person), or sometimes there may only be a single strong CEO (some Israeli models). Thus, the quest for a magic number may well be futile. Indeed, as the above-mentioned distribution implies, optimal board size is necessarily dependent on the broader institutional and external context. A second topic that has received considerable attention, diversity in board composition, can strengthen the board's decision-making capacity and legitimacy, particularly with external stakeholders; however, it also can be a potential drawback in that it can increase conflict and slow down decision-making. Overall, some diversity in board members' tenure, gender, and professional and educational backgrounds seems intuitively valuable.

4.2.5 Governing hospitals in a continuum of care

In order to accommodate the hospital's changed context, governance models should no longer be realistically considered to be either linear or political in nature, but rather as reflecting the melted boundaries and functional orientation that now characterize the entire care continuum in health service delivery. Hospital governance in this new context becomes focused on steering one or several elements within a new network, rather than (as before) assuming a free-standing and wholly separate institution. The considerable variation between (and sometimes within) countries provides a natural laboratory through which the overall benefits of different models can be assessed. Both aspects of this new situation help highlight for policy-makers the strategic and/or operational advantages and disadvantages of adopting hospital organization and governance models in the future. Among the most interesting – and most controversial – questions in this new functional context are the following

1. A key issue is what the future will be likely to hold – for example, where the current interplay of dynamics is taking these changed governance modalities. Will the new models of governance be extended to all public hospitals? Or will some of these new models slip away in the future, back into more traditional political control? How sustainable are these new models over the short and medium term? Are they digging deeper roots, or are they likely to fade in importance? What can be done to make them more sustainable?

2. What actually happens in practice rather than the formal rules for governing these new hospital models? Officially, major elements of control are to be transferred from politically led actors to professional managers and to a new set of Supervisory Boards. To what extent does that actually

happen? What new, complex relationships between old and new forms of governance end up being worked out? To what extent do these new hospital models find themselves sliding back over time into more direct political and/or public sector union control?

3. Taken overall, what have been/are the advantages and disadvantages of developing these new governance processes and tools? To what extent has it been a worthwhile endeavour?

4. Have the new models performed better or worse than the straight politically managed versions that they supersede? How different is the performance of the new meso-level governance arrangements on key parameters, such as clinical, managerial and financial? Are they measurably better than their fully politically managed public sector peers? To what extent have the new models affected patient issues or equity (social and geographic)?

This volume tries to provide at least some initial responses to the first three of these questions. The fourth one has been left open for a future study to address. Such a study would require a credible conceptual framework that can generate correspondingly credible metrics.

4.3 Remaining issues

Beyond the general sense in most of the case study countries that the introduction of these new governance models for public hospitals has been worth the effort, there still remain a number of issues regarding the structure and behaviour of these models that have yet to be satisfactorily resolved.

1. Should these new models be placed under public or private law? In several regions in Spain, new hospitals have been placed under private law, as a means of unencumbering them from the entrenched bureaucratic (and expensive) patterns of traditional public sector hospital governance. In Estonia, and for some institutions in the Czech Republic, hospitals have also been placed under private law. In both these countries, these institutions remain publicly owned and publicly accountable; however, they are managed daily under the same criteria that define how private business operates.

2. Have the new models made unnecessary the privatization of public hospitals, and/or the growth and expansion of new private hospitals that could threaten the social cohesion created by a public hospital system? This is a crucial issue for the long-term legitimacy and sustainability of public hospital systems generally; however, it also is difficult to demonstrate empirically.

3. Does patient choice of public hospitals (or of public versus private, as is now the case in England) influence the development and sustainability of this new governance model? If these new model hospitals are better able to provide citizens with the timeliness and standard of care that they prefer, then perhaps these new models have the ability to attract more patients into, (or to retain more patients within), the public hospital system. Again, this is a hard question for which to obtain reliable data.

In the future it will be useful to review evidence regarding these and other analytical dimensions of these new governance approaches. In some cases, these new models were the intentional design of a government, and were put in place largely as they were conceived – Norway's state enterprise approach, for example, as well as England's Foundation Trusts. In other cases, the models evolved from a set of incremental needs, and were themselves incremental in nature – the five different approaches in Spain appear to have this character. In a third type of case, the original reform model did not work as expected; consequently a new strategy was developed at national level – here, one thinks of England in replacing Self-governing Trusts with the more recent concept of the Foundation Trusts, also Portugal replacing hospitals which were designated as "public companies" in 2002, but which have subsequently been transformed into PEEHs from 2005.

Ultimately, whether planned, incrementally evolved or a hybrid of these two approaches, it will be important to obtain better data relating to how these models have behaved on a variety of indices.

4.4 References

Bloom N et al. (2010). *Why good practices really matter in healthcare*. London, VoxEU.org, Centre for Economic Policy and Research (http://www.voxeu.org/index.php?q=node/5939, accessed 2 May 2011).

Harding A, Preker AS, eds. (2003). *Private participation in health services*. Washington, DC, World Bank.

Jessop B (1995). The regulation approach and governance theory: alternative perspectives on economic and political change. *Economy and Society*, 24(3): 307–333.

Jeurissen P (2010). *For-profit hospitals* [doctoral thesis]. Rotterdam, Erasmus University Rotterdam Press.

Saltman RB (1985). Power and cost containment in a Danish public hospital. *Journal of Health Politics, Policy and Law*, 9:563–594.

Saltman RB, Busse R (2002). Balancing regulation and entrepreneurialism in Europe's health sector: theory and practice. In: Saltman RB, Busse R, Mossialos E, eds. *Regulating entrepreneurial behaviour in European health care systems*. Buckingham, Open University Press:3–52.

Saltman RB, de Roo AA (1989). Hospital policy in the Netherlands: the parameters of structural stalemate. *Journal of Health Politics Policy and Law*, 14:773–795.

Vaillencourt-Rosenau P (2003). Performance evaluations of for-profit and non-profit US hospitals since 1980. *Non-profit Management and Leadership*, 13(4):401–422.

Weisbrod B (1988). *The non-profit economy*. Cambridge, MA, Harvard University Press.

Young DW, Saltman RB (1985). *The hospital power equilibrium: physician behavior and cost control*. Baltimore, MD, Johns Hopkins University Press.

Eight case studies: case study responses to key governance questions

Czech Republic

	Limited liability company	Joint-stock companies	Semi-budgetary organizations ("public contributory organizations")
Status/recognition	Owned by regional governments or municipalities as limited liability company. Portfolio negotiated with insurance fund. Ability to outsource. Staff mainly salaried, also self-employed.	Owned by regional governments as joint-stock company. Portfolio negotiated with insurance fund. Staff mainly salaried, also self-employed.	Owned by regional governments. Portfolio negotiated with insurance fund. Salaried staff.
Financing	Payment by the insurance funds. Manage cash flow and pay providers. Regional government may allow them to retain surpluses. Investments: regional government plus own sources, loans.	Payment by the insurance funds. Manage cash flow and pay providers. Regional government may allow them to retain surpluses. Investments: regional government plus own sources, loans.	Payment by the insurance funds. Manage cash flow and pay providers. Not allowed to retain surpluses. Investments: regional government.
Accountability	Supervisory Board appointed by regional government. Medium accountability. Meetings not open to the public. Reporting obligations as per commercial legislation.	Supervisory Board appointed by regional government. Medium accountability. Meetings not open to the public. Reporting obligations as per commercial legislation.	Board of Trustees appointed by regional government. Meetings not open to the public. No specific reporting obligations.
Decision capacity versus responsibility	Medium political interference. Difficult for managers to change professional structures but proposals possible. Information shared with staff.	Medium political interference. Difficult for managers to change professional structures but proposals possible. Information shared with staff.	Political interference. Virtually impossible for managers to change professional structures.

England

	Foundation Trusts	Self-governing Trusts (expected to be abolished)
Status/recognition	Licensed by the regulator (Monitor) after achieving Foundation Trust status. Monitor specifies services, high-level discretion beyond that. Need to consult extensively. Staff mostly salaried. Freedom to change staff terms and conditions.	Statutory organizations dependent on Secretary of State for Health. Some decision on services portfolio, despite more constraints from regional authorities. Central negotiation of pay and conditions of employment. Nationally set pay scales.
Financing	Revenues from purchaser; do retain surpluses; asset disposal. May borrow from banks (up to 2014, Monitor sets limits and signs off borrowing regime) or Foundation Trust Financing Facility. Very large capital financed through private patient partnership (currently underwritten by Department of Health). Foundation Trust Board with complete freedom to invest.	No commercial borrowing. Financed from allocations by the government and purchaser. May retain surpluses; asset disposal. Internal deployment of revenue generated. Large capital through private patient partnerships or central government capital funds. Should aim to break even over three years.
Accountability	Board of Governors elected by the members (patients, staff and public). Non-executives plus a chair approved by the Board of Governors. No regional authority involvement. Monitor has powers to intervene. Scrutiny by local governments. No obligation for public meetings, but some Foundation Trusts do. Commercial law insolvency regime.	Board appointed by independent commission and the Trust. Executives appointed by the Board. Regional involvement in CEO appointments. Political intervention in strategic decisions (not operational matters). Scrutiny by local government. Meetings in public.
Decision capacity versus responsibility	Boards have high level of discretion and are accountable for their decisions (roughly free from political interference). Free to affect professional structures (only a few internal operational posts mandated). Some mandatory reporting.	High level of decision-making autonomy but can be overruled and influenced by regional authorities. Free to affect professional structures (only a few internal operational posts mandated). Some mandatory reporting.

Estonia

	Joint-stock company	Foundation
Status/recognition	Owned by national and municipal governments as shareholders, subject to commercial law. Basic portfolio decided by Ministry of Social Affairs in the context of government Hospital Master Plan (HMP); introduction of new services needs government approval. Most staff contracted; some self-employed.	Owned by founder(s) (public institutions), subject to Foundations Act. Basic portfolio decided by the Ministry of Social Affairs in the context of government HMP; introduction of new services needs government approval. Most staff contracted; some self-employed.
Financing	Most revenue from activity-based contracts negotiated between the hospital and the Estonian Health Insurance Fund (EHIF) on service volume and service mix; additionally, co-payments for ambulatory specialists and limited hospital bed days. Hospital can retain surpluses and is responsible for deficits. Capital financed from loans and EU structural fund grants.	Most revenue from activity-based contracts negotiated between the hospital and the EHIF on service volume and mix of services; additionally, co-payments for ambulatory specialists and limited hospital bed days. Hospital can retain surpluses and is responsible for deficits. Capital financed from loans and EU structural fund grants.
Accountability	Supervisory Board appointed by shareholders (with representation of national/ municipal governments as owners). Management Board appointed by Supervisory Board. No patient involvement – board meetings not open to public. Obligation to publish annual reports.	Supervisory Board appointed by shareholders (with representation of national/ municipal governments as founders). CEO appointed by Supervisory Board; Management Board members either appointed by CEO or by Supervisory Board. No patient involvement – board meetings not open to public. Obligation to publish annual reports.
Decision capacity versus responsibility	Supervisory Board could be overpoliticized. Management can affect professional and internal operational structures. Decision-making power delegated to units ("clinics").	Supervisory Board could be overpoliticized. Management can affect professional and internal operational structures. Decision-making power delegated to units ("clinics").

Israel

	Government owned	Private non-profit-making	Sick fund owned	Private, sick fund major shareholder
Status/recognition	Public asset as per general law. Service portfolio by Ministry of Health; planning ratified by Board of Directors and hospital management. Staff subject to national salary agreements.	United States-based private company. Service portfolio by hospital management and Board of Directors, subject to Ministry of Health approval. Staff subject to national salary agreements.	Sick fund-owned private company. Service portfolio by hospital management and regional and national sick fund, subject to Ministry of Health approval. Staff subject to national salary agreements.	Private company. Service portfolio by hospital management and Board of Directors subject to Ministry of Health approval. Staff contracted. No unionization.
Financing	Capped targeted hospital activities (tariff reductions above cap). Can retain surpluses. "Extra" services for privately arranged and/or supplemental insurance policies (patient payments to "research funds", formally not for choice). Capital investment by government (Ministry of Health/Ministry of Finance/ parliamentary approval) and "friendly" organizations. Specific investment decisions by management, subject to Ministry of Health approval.	Capped targeted hospital activities (tariff reductions above cap). Can retain surpluses. Patient choice if paid for out of pocket or by supplemental insurance (subject to strict physician/hospital income sharing arrangements). Capital investment by owners with own funds, bank loans, etc. Specific investment decisions by management, subject to Board of Directors' and Ministry of Health approval.	Prospective budgets from regional and national sick fund offices (taking into account other sick funds' behaviour). Income from capped targeted hospital activities (tariff reductions above cap). Can retain surpluses (prior to authorization of sick fund). Capital investment from national and regional sick fund and "friendly" organizations. Investment decisions by management (prior authorization of regional and/or national sick fund headquarters).	Block contracts with sick funds plus private pay, based on supplemental insurance, private insurance and direct out-of-pocket payments. Can retain surpluses. Capital investment by shareholders with own funds, bank loans, etc. Specific investment decisions by Director, with Board approval.

Israel (cont.)

	Government owned	Private non-profit-making	Sick fund owned	Private, sick fund major shareholder
Accountability	Direct control by Ministry of Health (must supply data on patient flows, medical mishaps and salaried employees). State controller evaluates hospital performance. No Supervisory Board or direct citizen participation.	Owners, a number of seats on Board of Directors; additional members proposed by management and approved by owners. Owner-appointed *controller* (reporting to them) plus *State controller* who officially evaluates hospital performance. No Supervisory Board, no direct citizen participation.	Hospital director reports to sick fund headquarters; members and Labor Federation Members with indirect access through *forums*. State controller evaluates hospital performance. No Supervisory Board. Need to report to Ministry of Health patient flows and medical mishaps.	Board of Directors elected by shareholders. No Supervisory Board or direct citizen participation, but need to report to Ministry of Health on patient flows and medical mishaps.
Decision capacity versus responsibility	Direct political influence. Management has little or no control over workforce costs. Freedom to partially affect professional and internal operational structures (subject to Ministry of Health requirements).	Medium level of political interference. Management has little or no control over workforce costs. Can affect professional and internal operational structures (subject to Ministry of Health requirements).	Limited by instructions of regional and/or national sick fund headquarters. Management has little or no control over workforce costs. Can affect professional and internal operational structures (only subject to Ministry of Health and fund headquarters requirements).	Near-complete autonomy for hospital management to achieve the goals set by the Board. Freedom to affect professional and internal operational structures.

Netherlands

	Private non-profit-making foundations
Status/recognition	All hospitals are non-profit-making foundations. Profit-making hospitals are not allowed by law. Hospitals require a government licence to provide services. Due to the market reform, hospital decisions on the service portfolio are no longer subject to Ministry of Health approval. Staff: 30% salaried (with employee contracts and subordinated to the Executive Board) and 70% self-employed (fee-for-service payments).
Financing	Case-based hospital funding (fixed tariff for each variant (numerous) of a DRG system using so-called diagnosis–treatment combinations (DTCs). Able to retain surpluses and has to bear the deficits if they occur. Capital financing by borrowing from banks.
Accountability	Supervisory Board appointed by cooptation (but increasingly selected on the basis of expertise), without political involvement (appointments by Ministry of Health, Welfare and Sport only in exceptional circumstances). Executive Board appointed by Supervisory Board (but Employees' Council and Clients' Council can give opinion on appointments). Executive Board sets overall budget estimates, which Supervisory Board approves. Required to publish an annual Financial Account and an annual quality of care account. Board meetings not open to public. Citizen participation through the Clients' Council.
Decision capacity versus responsibility	Almost totally free from political interference (but Ministry of Health, Welfare and Sport intervention in exceptional cases). Hospital divisions and units with their own budget and management – high discretionary managerial power. Executive Board's control over physicians is weak, particularly in the case of self-employed physicians.

Norway

	Independent health trust (used interchangeably with "hospital", although an independent health trust may contain more than one hospital)
Status/recognition	Explicitly independent legal entities with governing bodies and annual general assembly (similar to private firms). Owned by regional health authorities and regulated by statutes; reflecting central instructions, each regional health authority gives annual governing instructions (budget allocation and expected "balanced budget", investments, overall goals related to activity and quality, etc.). Service portfolio decided by regional health authorities (most hospitals need to buy certain services from other hospitals). Private sector may establish facilities, but need to contract with regional health authorities. Employees are remunerated by means of fixed salaries, primarily set through national negotiations.
Financing	Dual financial governance. Hospital budget as a combination of estimated relative need of catchment population and actual activity (reflecting the combination of capitation and activity-based income of the regional health authorities). Capital framework set out by the regional health authorities (50% of total investment costs transferred from special grants by Ministry of Health and Care Services and the remaining 50% coming from accumulated surpluses in the regional health authorities).
Accountability	Hospital ("local") board appointed by the regional health authorities, in turn appointed by the Ministry of Health. Includes politicians; some regional health authorities place their own representative as chairman of the board but it can also be an external appointee. No direct citizen involvement in decision-making, but board meetings open to the public. Every regional health authorities has a full-time appointed ombudsman. Reporting on goals is compulsory. Information provided (mostly monthly, some even on weekly basis) depending on the organizational level at the receiving end. Capital costs explicitly included in hospital accounting.
Decision capacity versus responsibility	Local health trusts are formally autonomous and able to decide on internal institutional arrangements, financial arrangements and, to some extent, accountability arrangements, including those affecting professional and internal operational structures. Staff hiring and purchase of equipment decisions (budgets) allocated according to levels of responsibility. Yet, hospitals have rather small overall autonomy: key decisions regarding investment, location and size of the facilities — "redrawing" the organizational map of the hospital, etc. — are made by regional health authorities (less direct interference from Ministry of Health and Care Services).

Portugal

	PEEHs	Administrative Public Sector Hospitals (APSH)
Status/recognition	Ownership public. Generic statute for all PEEHs. State (the "custody", represented by Ministry of Finance and Ministry of Health) as main shareholder. In practice, little room to define service portfolio (including setting up private clinical practices within the hospital, which is possible), need permission from Ministry of Health. Staff allowed to opt for employment contract (labour contracts or public servants). May contract with private physicians for specific individual services.	Ownership public. Generic Statute for APSHs. Staff made of public servants.
Financing	Financial framework defined in the statute. A total of 80% of revenues from state budget funding within National Framework Contract Programme – mainly based on previous year's funding, adjusted for inflation but a growing fraction based on DRGs and non-adjusted hospital outpatient volumes. Additional revenues from payments for special services, private insurance, and law-defined user charges for outpatient and diagnostic services. Hospital can retain surpluses. Capital investments financed from annual budgets, grants, private donations and loans. Free to invest up to 2% of statutory capital; free commercial borrowing up to 10% of statutory capital – Ministry of Finance and Ministry of Health approval needed beyond that.	A total of 80% of revenues from state budget-funded contract, framed by the National Framework Contract Programme. Budget mainly based on previous year's funding, updated for inflation plus growing fraction based on DRGs and on non-adjusted hospital outpatient volumes.
Accountability	No Board of Trustees. Administration Board appointed by Ministry of Health and Ministry of Finance (may include a non-executive member proposed by the municipality). Upwardly accountable to Ministry of Health and Ministry of Finance. Meetings not open to public. Monthly report on clinical and financial performance. Must use the Official Accounting Plan of the Ministry of Health (OAPMH). Annual Report to be approved by Ministry of Finance and Ministry of Health.	As per national civil service specifications.
Decision capacity versus responsibility	Intense political interference. Some formal freedom to affect professional structures but very limited effective capacity of management to implement decisions outside politically driven goals.	As per national civil service specifications.

Spain

	Public Healthcare Company	Public Healthcare Foundation	Foundation	Consortium	Administrative Concession
Status/recognition	Regional law. Portfolio by regional health department. Non-statutory staff.	Secondary legislation. Portfolio by regional health department. Statutory staff.	Secondary legislation. Partially decide on services portfolio. Non-statutory staff.	Agreements with non-profit-making organization. Decide on services portfolio. Non-statutory staff.	Contract with private company. Partially decide on portfolio. Non-statutory and statutory staff.
Financing	Capital investment under public procurement law. Budget. Not able to retain surpluses.	Capital investment under public procurement law. Budget. Not able to retain surpluses.	Free to invest; for high-volume contracts, procurement law. Manage cash flow and pay providers. Can retain surpluses but need to reinvest in hospital.	Free to invest; for high-volume contracts, procurement law. Activity and capitation payment. Manage cash flow. Can retain surpluses but need to reinvest.	Free to decide sources of capital investment and not subject to national procurement law. Capitation. Can retain surpluses. Overall profit capped.
Accountability	Supervisory Board chaired by regional health minister. No patient involvement. No reporting obligations.	Supervisory Board partially appointed by regional health minister. No patient involvement. No reporting obligations.	Supervisory Board chaired by regional health minister. No patient involvement. Accounts registered annually.	Supervisory Board of participating organizations. Local business people on the Board. Annual report.	Management Board, Joint Committee and Commissioner. No patient involvement. Annual report.
Decision capacity versus responsibility	Intense political interference. Information partially shared with staff. Some freedom for clinical managers.	Intense political interference. Information partially shared with staff. Some freedom for clinical managers.	Intense political interference. Information partially shared with staff. Some freedom for clinical managers.	Low level of political interference. Information partially shared with staff. Some freedom for clinical managers.	Low level of political interference. Information partially shared with staff. Some freedom for clinical managers.

PART II
Hospital governance in eight countries

Chapter 5
Czech Republic

Tomas Roubal and Pavel Hroboň

5.1 Introduction

The Czech Republic has a system of SHI based on compulsory membership of every citizen in one of several non-profit-making health insurance funds, which are quasi-independent public bodies that act as payers and purchasers of care. The system is financed primarily through SHI contributions in the form of a mandatory payroll tax administered by the health insurance funds; other sources of funding are general taxation and out-of-pocket payments (Bryndová et al., 2009).

The basic benefits package covered by SHI in the Czech Republic is very broad and includes nearly all services that are not mentioned in the negative list, regulated by law (Mátl et al., 2008).

In 2008, the Czech Republic had 192 acute-care hospitals with 63 622 beds, 10.3% of which were dedicated to long-term patient care. There were also 154 other inpatient facilities with 22 191 beds, 42% of which were in psychiatric care and 32% of which were in long-term care. Of the 192 hospitals, 25 were owned by the central state (30% of beds), 66 were owned by the regions (46% of beds), and 28 were owned by the municipalities (7.5% of beds). There were 12 hospitals with over 1000 beds and 30 hospitals with fewer than 100 beds. In comparative international terms, the number of physicians in the Czech Republic is rather high, with 3.6 physicians per 1000 population in 2007. The nurse-to-population ratio is above the averages for the EU15[10] and the EU10[11] (Bryndová et al., 2009).

---

10 Countries belonging to the EU before May 2004.

11 Countries that joined the EU in May 2004.

The regional authorities are responsible for registering hospitals and other health care facilities that are not owned or operated by the central state (that is, the private practices of nearly all providers of outpatient care, as well as the majority of inpatient providers). A variety of laws and regulations define the technical, staffing and hygienic requirements that all providers must fulfil in order to be permitted to supply health care services. Non-state providers may provide health services only once they have been registered by the relevant regional authority.

5.2 Historical background

In the early 1990s, the system changed radically from a Soviet-type NHS system to the SHI model described in the previous section. Up to 25 new insurance funds emerged during the 1990s, some of which went bankrupt or merged together – there are currently eight insurance funds. The first health insurance fund to be established was the General Health Insurance Fund (VZP), the largest health insurance fund in the Czech Republic since its founding in early 1992. It has the biggest influence due to its market share and its function as a safety net for members of health insurance funds that close down or go bankrupt.

During the 1990s, changes made to the structure of inpatient facilities in the Czech Republic were driven primarily by an excessive number of beds in acute care and an insufficient number of beds in long-term care. A variety of measures were taken by the Czech central government in the first half of the 1990s to address this situation, including closing small, redundant inpatient facilities or restructuring them into long-term care facilities. These early measures were generally successful, leading to a rapid fall in the number of acute-care beds, as well as to a sharp rise in the acute-care bed occupancy rate between 1992 and 2000.

After the year 2000, hospital restructuring focused more on specialization. Instead of closing entire hospitals, hospital owners began to close or merge individual departments, while the transformation of smaller acute-care hospitals into long-term nursing care and rehabilitation facilities continued. Again, these developments resulted primarily from the decisions made by the facilities' owners and were not of an explicitly political nature. With the exception of inpatient facilities directly subordinate to the Ministry of Health, a considerable number of hospitals – including some in regional ownership – underwent this process of rationalization (Bryndová et al., 2009).

5.3 Public administration reform

In 1998, the Czech Republic began a far-reaching process of decentralization in public administration. Over the course of five years, executive power was gradually devolved from state-administered districts to 14 newly formed regions. This has had important consequences for the administration of hospitals and other public health care facilities.

Before 2003, most hospitals in the Czech Republic were owned by the state and operated by state-administered districts (*okresy*). However, state administration at the district level was abolished at the end of 2002 and replaced by a system of regional governments (*kraje*). Although almost half of the hospitals in the country were subsequently transferred into regional ownership, some smaller hospitals are now owned and operated by municipalities, and several dozen others have been privatized. Most of the hospitals in regional ownership have been converted into joint-stock companies, which as of 2010 are still owned entirely by the regions and continue to be financed primarily through contracts with the health insurance funds.

The public administration reform was the main incentive for the change of legal form of many hospitals. It also caused a change of owner of the two hospitals in this case study. The public administration reform was part of the process of transition from the communist type of public governance into the democratic form of public governance. It began in 1990, when public governance duties were centralized. On the one hand this enabled a smooth political transformation, including organizing the first free elections. On the other hand, it centralized too many competences at the central level, which caused many problems relating to the coordination and implementation of new laws and regulations. So the next step was to create a new municipal and regional system of governance. Based on the new constitutional law of 1997, the principle of subsidiarity was defined. This law defined the competences and responsibilities of each of the layers involved in public governance (central, regional, municipal).

The first phase of the new public administration system was the creation of 14 regions. The second phase was abolition of districts and the transfer of their competences and property to the newly established regions and also to the municipalities. These steps were also in line with the *acquis communautaire*, the adoption of which is a prerequisite for joining the EU (in 2004).

In summary, this transition was part of the larger process started in 1989, and the change of ownership of hospitals previously owned by districts was just a by-product of this process. The district hospital represented the largest group of hospitals in 2001 (81), having the highest number of beds (49.6%) and hospitalizations (51.4%), as well as employing the most workers (45.7%). However, the overall negative trend of poor economic results continued.

The issue of management of hospitals came to the fore in connection with the transfer of district hospitals to the regions, where the new founders became concerned about the financial state of these facilities. It emerged that the deficit has led in many hospitals to failure to fulfil obligations to suppliers, which in late 2002 produced a threat from pharmaceutical distributors to stop supplies. As a result, improving the efficiency of these facilities became a central task for the new owner.

The previous owner of these hospitals (the Czech central Government) paid Czech koruna (CZK) 2.7 billion to cover the bad debts of these hospitals, thereby improving their financial situation and cash flow. The government also transferred CZK 3 billion to the health insurance funds to enable them to increase their reimbursements to providers.

Hospital governance is limited by the level of regulation and depends very much on the position of the hospital within the whole health care sector. The payers – that is, the insurance funds – should play the most important role in terms of allocating money and purchasing care according to patient needs, as well as in provider efficiency and quality. However, historically they have been set up only as distributers of premiums into various health care segments and they did not play a major role in purchasing services for their clients. This was also caused by relatively strict regulation by the Ministry of Health. The situation has been changing only slowly in recent years (Roubal, 2009).

The entire health system is negatively influenced by the lack of a clear vision based on societal agreement. There are rapid and considerable changes caused by political turnover. This creates a difficult playing field for hospital management to plan and govern the facilities.

The Ministry of Health is currently introducing the centralization of highly specialized services into selected facilities that will provide the most advanced care in oncology, cardiology, traumatology and cerebrovascular diseases. This development is spurred by structural funds from the EU that are being invested into new technologies and equipment. Insurance funds transfer the financial flows into these new centres and do not purchase these advanced procedures and services from non-designated hospitals. This has caused the loss of some "profitable" procedures, as well as a decrease in reimbursement for non-designated hospitals. These changes are slowly disrupting the balance in the hospital system and there is a small but persistent push for hospitals to close some wards. This strategy is new and it will be interesting to follow its effects.

Regulation by the Ministry of Health does not fully cover the continuity of care between the centres of excellence and the rest of health care providers. Since neither of the hospitals in this case study is a designated centre, they both have to cope with some decrease in reimbursement, as well as accepting patients who still need follow-up care from such centres (which is not particularly profitable). The Czech system does not allow any managerial right to refuse such patients, as patients can choose their provider and the provider is required to accept them.

5.4 Legal forms of ownership in health care in the Czech Republic

In the Czech Republic, there is no legislation generally defining non-profit-making organizations. Nearly all health care establishments and companies claim to be non-profit-making organizations; however, for this to be the case, they must be based on some existing legal form, defined in legislation. The most common legal forms are semi-budgetary organization, joint-stock company and limited liability company.

According to the law, the commercial legal form of a company is established mainly for business purposes, but may exist (based on the decision of the owner) in a not-for-profit form as well. The most common legal forms in health care are limited liability companies and joint-stock companies. During the transformation process of the whole economy in the Czech Republic, these legal forms were significantly improved so that they have clearly defined their corporate bodies (Board of Directors, Supervisory Board, Annual Meeting, etc.) and the corresponding governance mechanisms through which the owner controls the organization. The roles and responsibilities are clear and the accounting, tax and legal standards of operation are transparent. The legislation is fairly similar to that of other developed countries, but the semi-budgetary organization, which is subject to public law, needs to be described in more detail.

In 1990, all hospitals were owned by the state in the form of budgetary organizations (legal form defined since 1952). The regional structure of health care authorities from the communist era was abandoned in the early part of 1990. Some smaller hospitals and nearly all outpatient providers (including pharmacies) were privatized. The remaining hospitals were transformed into semi-budgetary organizations, owned by the state through district administrations or municipalities. The budgetary organization form of ownership was completely abandoned in the year 2000.

With the reform of the public administration system in 2003, district hospitals were automatically transferred to regional authorities. Regional hospitals which have not been transformed into joint-stock companies or limited liability companies (as was Hospital Kadaň, described in the following sections) continue to exist as semi-budgetary organizations (as has Hospital Jablonec nad Nisou) – a change of legal form aiming to improve some of the shortcomings of semi-budgetary organizations, namely low accountability, transparency and managerial responsibility.

5.5 Semi-budgetary organizations (*příspěvková organizace*)

A semi-budgetary organization is a Czech form of legal entity that can be established by a governmental body, to which the entity's budget is linked. The name of the organization was defined as a form of ownership in the 1960s and implies some subsidies to be transferred from the owner to the organization. The semi-budgetary organization's main rationale was to perform various tasks in public interest (museums, libraries, galleries, schools, shelters for animals, etc.) and they also receive revenue from other sources, rather than just subsidies (hence the term semi-budgetary).

A semi-budgetary organization is according to the law created by a Deed of Foundation. The founder and owner appoint and dismiss its director, decide on her/his remuneration, can file a complaint against her/him and control the finances of the entire organization. The Deed must contain the name, define the major and secondary activities of the organization, delegate the director and define the property rights between the owner and the organization. Thus, the director is the only body of the semi-budgetary organization defined by law. No other bodies are created (as is also the case with limited liability companies and joint-stock companies) and the director's status is that of an employee.

The main benefit of a semi-budgetary organization is the simplicity of control for the owner. The organization has to comply with rules regarding the level of wages centrally set by the government (although there is significant room for upwards flexibility, in the event that the financial situation of an organization allows for such an adjustment). However, the director is the only one with all competences; control bodies are not defined; there are no rules set; and no control mechanism is defined, which creates a grey area in which owners can enforce their own will. In general, there is a low level of transparency; the organization is not particularly well suited for tax optimization, and there often are problems in terms of accountancy and other aspects of company management.

5.6 Hospitals studied: Hospital Jablonec nad Nisou, p.o. and Hospital Kadaň s.r.o

It is possible to identify examples of hospitals which have developed successfully in this often unpredictable climate and have developed a set of experiences and tools which helped them to fulfil new expectations.

We have chosen two cases, with two different approaches to the development of a hospital in the same environment within the Czech health care system. Both the studied hospitals are owned by a municipality and are regarded by their peers as well-run institutions. Moreover, both of them had to adapt to competition from a nearby, larger hospital run by the regional administration. One of them decided (Hospital Jablonec nad Nisou) to keep the form of a semi-budgetary organization. The other one (Hospital Kadaň) transformed quite early in its development to a limited liability company, but remained fully owned by the municipality.

The hospital in Jablonec nad Nisou is a regional hospital in the northern part of the Czech Republic. Currently, the hospital provides health services in 16 medical specialties across 310 acute-care beds and 67 long-term care beds. The hospital has 695 employees (of which 99 physicians and 353 nurses). In 2008, there were 14 800 hospitalized patients, with an average length of stay of seven days. Over 6000 surgeries were performed and there were 1329 births. In 1991 the Hospital Jablonec nad Nisou became a state semi-budgetary organization. The owner was the district authority of Jablonec nad Nisou. After the public administration reform, the ownership of the hospital was handed over to the municipality of the town Jablonec nad Nisou from 1 March 2003, but the legal form was retained as a semi-budgetary organization.

The hospital in Kadaň is a small local hospital in the western part of the Czech Republic. Currently, the hospital provides services in 9 medical specialties across 200 acute-care beds and 30 long-term care beds. The hospital has 362 employees. In 2009, there were 9400 hospitalized patients with an average length of stay of 5.6 days. Over 2600 surgeries were performed and there were nearly 800 births. Before 1989, the hospital in Kadaň was part of the district system of public health care facilities and, thanks to its proximity to the western border of one of the largest military areas in the middle of Europe (Vojenský újezd Hradiště), the planned capacity was much higher than current needs. At the beginning of the 1990s, the hospital was transformed into a semi-budgetary organization owned by the district (*okresní úřad*). During the public administration reform, the hospital became a semi-budgetary organization of the region, which was immediately brought under the municipality of Kadaň, which adjusted the legal form of the hospital to a limited liability company in January 2004.

5.7 Comparison of the hospitals studied

The final decision regarding the legal form of the hospital was in both cases based on the regional experience and the political situation concerned. The municipality of Kadaň had good experience with organizational governance in the form of limited liability companies. Moreover, the director of the Kadaň hospital was a member of the municipal council and was, therefore, better positioned to influence the transformation. At the other end of the scale, the municipality of Jablonec nad Nisou did not have much experience with commercial legal forms of ownership and chose to continue with the semi-budgetary organization legal form.

The main difference between the hospitals studied is the governance and accountability framework within which the management operates. As already anticipated, whereas the hospital in Kadaň – run as a limited liability company – has well-defined control bodies and a standard accounting system, the semi-budgetary organization hospital in Jablonec nad Nisou is controlled by a director and a hospital board. However, the board is a voluntary establishment without any legal definition and does not take any responsibility for the conduct of the hospital and decisions made. Full responsibility lies with the director.

Although the two legal forms are quite different, the directors of both hospitals have significant scope for governance. They bear full responsibility for their actions towards the owners of the hospitals and they have the power to decide on matters relating to the structural and institutional frameworks concerned. They created a motivated team of managers who help them with their day-to-day decisions.

The most challenging task for the management was to change the mindset of all employees who had become used to different motivation, under the previous hospital governance set-up. The wages were mostly uniform – regardless of how hard they tried (or did not) to change this – during the communist era. The middle management was not aware of the costs and revenues generated by their wards, even during the 1990s. Their compensation was not dependent on the economic situation of the hospital. In the event of any financial problems, the state (via district authorities) subsidized the organization. This attitude was quite deeply rooted in employees of all levels and the management knew that this had to change in order for the new governance models to succeed.

One of the most successful management tools was to directly connect wages and other benefits of employees with the performance of individual wards and the whole hospital. The management of the Hospital Jablonec nad Nisou divided the hospital into several parts, which act as individual producers and "sell" their services to other parts within the hospital. Every part receives a financial and health care plan for the coming year from the management. Successfully fulfilling the plan is directly connected with the bonuses that are available, which is a good motivator for production. Three times a year the management holds a discussion and presents results in every ward.

The Hospital Kadaň also prepares plans for its wards, which are connected with financial bonuses for employees. Moreover, the management carries out benchmarking of its performance within and outside the hospital. There is a special team in every ward that meets on a weekly basis to assess all expensive or atypical treated cases, looking for inefficiencies and identifying best practices. Based on this assessment, the management can choose to increase some activities or decrease them if the results are not satisfactory over a longer period.

The change in mindset is believed to be more effective if employees are allowed to find the best solution themselves, without much direct management. This is why neither hospital enforces formal positive lists. However, every ward has a budget of material, pharmaceuticals and other medical supplies. The management of both hospitals created a special unit, the task of which is to monitor and prepare overviews of pricing related to pharmaceuticals, medical supplies and materials, for the attention of the middle management of each ward. Based on the preferences of the matron and head physician, a decision is made regarding what to buy. More expensive materials consume a larger part of the budget and decrease financial bonuses.

5.7.1 Leadership

From the authors' perspective, the people in charge of leading the hospitals are the main reason for the success of the hospitals studied. Their leadership and knowledge has enabled the flourishing of both hospitals in the Czech health care market.

The director of the Hospital Kadaň is one of the longest-serving directors of a hospital in the Czech Republic. He played a substantial role in the transition process of becoming a limited liability company.

Until 2002, no managerial tools were used in the hospital in Jablonec nad Nisou. This changed with the arrival of a new director, who in turn hired a manager – these two individuals still run the hospital today. They introduced the new managerial tools described in this study and their leadership has served to motivate the hospital's other employees.

5.7.2 Internal communication

As already mentioned, the hospital management in Jablonec nad Nisou organizes three meetings with each ward every year, at which they discuss the goals of the whole hospital and evaluate the ward's results from the previous and current years. The management also introduced structured interviews between the middle management tier and employees in an attempt to promote collaboration and mutual motivation. The hospital in Kadaň is very small, which means that the director works closely with the employees. Although his style is quite directive, he is highly respected within the hospital. The hospital in Kadaň uses its intranet to disseminate financial results and plans among employees, ensuring everyone has access to all necessary information.

The financial framework is prepared annually by the management teams in a very detailed manner, in both hospitals. Every ward has its own budget, with selected indicators (financial and health care production) to monitor its success.

As discussed before, the directors have a very high level of freedom to organize their hospitals' internal operating structures. This is mainly due to a high level of long-term trust which has been built between directors and owner (the municipal council). The hospital in Kadaň has mapped and monitored processes in detail, and has defined benchmarks and best practices. This is mainly due to the enthusiasm of the director for this kind of governance.

Communication with patients is also very intensive in both hospitals. The hospital in Jablonec nad Nisou provides its employees with coaching courses regarding communication with patients. Both hospitals have used patient satisfaction questionnaires since the early 2000s. The hospital in Jablonec nad Nisou has an external specialized agency, which carries out the patient satisfaction investigation. It consists not only of questionnaires but also observations, patient interviews and other sociological tools. The hospital in Kadaň also uses questionnaires, and patients can discuss directly their experiences with and address their remarks to the director. In both hospitals, patient satisfaction influences the remuneration of every ward and every employee.

5.7.3 Relationship with the owner and boards

In the hospitals studied, the board consists of political representatives of the owner and should thus represent the local community, public and patients simultaneously. The staff members sometimes use the labour unions to interfere with the management of the hospital.

The composition of the board or similar body does not seem principally important in the two hospitals studied. What is important is the relationship between the owner and the management. As long as the management achieves the basic (sometimes implicit) targets – financial sustainability, social stability, job security, high-quality services and positive public image – based on face-to-face interviews with the management of selected hospitals, the board composition is irrelevant. According to the hospitals studied, it is sometimes better when the board is inactive and does not influence managerial decisions, since the influencing of the running of the hospital by the board is believed to be mostly motivated by individual political or economic interests. There are examples from other hospitals in the Czech Republic in which board members used their power to outsource some profitable hospital services to favoured private companies.

The hospital managers are free to outsource some operations and it is their responsibility. As long as the hospital's economic results do not impact negatively the budget of the owner and do not interrupt political agreements, the owners have not restricted managers' autonomy in this field.

5.7.4 Investment policy

In both hospitals studied there are established rules for investment decisions. Up to a fixed sum of investment, the management is fully entitled to decide on such matters. Above this limit, the investment must be discussed with the owner. These investments are usually planned and the two hospitals studied plan such investments carefully, together with the owner.

The hospital in Jablonec nad Nisou has created a special committee that considers the investment alternatives. It also currently uses a new source of financing of investments – the European structural funds. Thanks to these funds, the hospital has been able to purchase magnetic resonance imaging (MRI) equipment. The management also enforces an "open book" policy, in which all selection procedures are public, including the offers and prices. This sets a high level of transparency and apparently also helps to obtain low prices.

5.7.5 Economic performance

The main sources of revenue are the insurance funds, subsidies from the owner, the regional authority and the central government. The (relatively) smallest revenue quantities are payments from patients and private donors.

The development of payments from insurance funds is relatively stable and there have been only minor changes recently (such as the possibility of a contract-defined number of total hip replacements for a defined price). One of the main changes in the financing of hospitals was connected with the change of ownership of the hospitals studied. As the municipalities took over the ownership of the hospitals, they realized that they did not have the financial means to subsidize the hospitals and the subsidies sharply decreased. In the hospital in Jablonec nad Nisou this had negative consequences and the financial loss in 2002 was over €1 000 000 (not taking into account the depreciation). Thanks to the managerial decisions described in this chapter, the hospital is currently in profit of around €1 000 000 (not taking into account the depreciation).

The hospital in Kadaň experienced a similar development: its operating result in 2003 was €–500 000 and it is currently €400 000. The positive results were also facilitated by the growth of the whole economy in the Czech Republic in recent years. The management will have to face further challenges in order to maintain such good economic results in the coming years of economic downturn.

5.7.6 Other questions

Q: Is there a particular type of auditing, or types and effects of different rules and regulations, that matter?

A: No, not in the hospitals studied. Hospitals studied use standard external auditing companies and produce annual reports that are available online. The hospital in Jablonec nad Nisou had to cooperate closely with an external auditing company when it faced many accountancy problems with the legal form associated with being a semi-budgetary organization.

Q: Is there a particular degree of managerial flexibility, in terms of contracting personnel, investments and so on?

A: There is quite considerable managerial flexibility in terms of contracting personnel, to the extent that it does not collide with the budget constraint, which is fairly strictly defined by the insurance funds and by governmental regulation.

Q: What is known about the relationship between governance and outcomes?

A: As far as financial outcomes are concerned, the high level of governance in the hospitals studied is demonstrated by their financial stability and their ability to adapt to a changing environment. As far as medical outcomes are concerned, there is no easy way to measure such a relationship. One interesting marker of high-quality services are the maternity and obstetrics wards. The delivery rates of these hospitals exceed their regional position in the spectrum of services. Pregnant women usually want to choose the best environment for their delivery and creating such conditions requires an active and innovative approach from hospital management.

5.8 Conclusions

Generally speaking, the change of legal status in itself did not lead to many changes in hospital governance or performance. It is also extremely difficult to separate changes due to new legal status from other local influences (e.g. politically motivated changes on the part of management) or country-wide influences (e.g. changes in the form of hospital payments or increases in payments to hospitals resulting from the better financial situation of the statutory health insurance system).

Moving ownership from state hands to the regions and the transformation to joint-stock companies owned by public entities have been just two milestones in a long process in which many hospitals in the Czech Republic since the early 1990s have moved from budgetary institutions to semi-autonomous status. These changes include (among others) responsibilities to negotiate contracts with payers within the statutory health insurance system, adaptation to new payment mechanisms, setting up internal control and motivation systems and managing relationships with a new, often inexperienced, owner.

5.9 References

Bryndová L et al. (2009). Czech Republic: health system review. *Health Systems in Transition*, 11(1):1–119.

Mátl O et al. (2008). *Zpráva o stavu, vývoji a výhledu zdravotnictví v ČR [Report on the state, development and perspective of health care in the Czech Republic]*. Prague, Kulatý stůl (http://www.kulatystul.cz/cs/system/files/Zprava+o+stavu_WEB.pdf, accessed 16 June 2011).

Roubal T (2009). New-fashioned instruments for changes in health care systems in the European countries. *Pojistné rozpravy*, 24.

Chapter 6
England

Nigel Edwards

6.1 Introduction: the current context

The English NHS is currently based on a quasi-market system with the following characteristics.

- Primary care gatekeeping: patients register with a primary care practice and are granted access to specialists through a referral system.

- A purchaser–provider split: Primary Care Trusts (PCTs) cover geographical areas of between 120 000 and 1 million people and are responsible for purchasing care and for health improvement. Increasingly payers (PCTs) delegate budgets to groups of general practitioners (GPs), who can act as purchasers for the services they use. It is intended that by 2013 the PCTs will be abolished and the payer function will be taken over by groups of GPs.

- Hospital reimbursement is largely carried out via an activity payment system based on casemix groups.

- Training, education and research: paid on a basis separate from hospital activity.

- National policy and direction: standards and policy objectives are set nationally.

- A more mixed economy for providers: the development of autonomous foundation hospitals and the encouragement of independent sector provision, especially in planned surgery.

- The NHS is now required to be much more transparent and accountable. Increasing amounts of information regarding providers is available publicly and Foundation Trust providers are required to produce a quality account alongside their financial statement and annual report. Standards are enforced by independent regulators, the scope and powers of which have greatly expanded since the early 2000s. In addition, patients now have legal rights to choice and maximum times for referral to treatment.

A theme of this book is the divergence between the legal and theoretical basis of hospital governance and experience in practice. In the United Kingdom, while there is often a significant gap between rhetoric and reality in public policy, and an important role for informal networks and local political influence, the formal rules that describe how hospital governance operates are quite close to what happens in reality.

This chapter looks at the experience of creating autonomous hospitals in the English NHS, how the governance arrangements have evolved and how they operate.

We have selected University College London Hospitals (UCLH) as the basis for a case study as it is a complex organization, serving a large number of payers and with an important role in research and education (see Box 6.2 in the following section). We have also been able to reference a small body of research and other material which allows more general conclusions to be drawn.

First, we present the history and background of the policy, which contains some important policy lessons. We then examine the main features of the model and its prospects for the future, including the early indications of further reforms following the election of a new government in May 2010, which will increase the level of autonomy given to providers.

6.2 The emergence of autonomous hospitals

6.2.1 Background

Compared with many other European systems, the English NHS is unusual in the extent to which the ownership and management of health care providers has been highly centralized and is government controlled (Box 6.1). Until the early 1990s, NHS hospitals and other providers were managed by health authorities, which were under the direct supervision of the central government. While they had their own management structures, they had little discretion over many important areas.

As a result of the Thatcher reforms in 1989, hospitals and other providers were allowed to apply to become self-governing organizations with some additional freedoms. During the 1990s, many of these freedoms were eroded, although in many cases the culture of the NHS had prevented some of them from being fully exercised (see Table 6.1). After Labour came to power in 1997, a resurgence of central control led to many freedoms being removed or discouraged.

Box 6.1 *Pre-1990 hospital governance*

- Pay and conditions determined by central government.
- Control of staff numbers for some staff groups – but not junior doctors, specialists and management.
- Specialist medical consultants appointed, employed and very rarely dismissed by regional authorities.
- Very limited discretion on capital spending. The largest capital schemes had to be approved by central government and even regional authorities had limited delegated powers.
- Global budgets set by district-level authorities, largely on an historic basis.
- Assets owned by central government.
- Large contracts had to be approved and were often drawn up at health authority or regional level.

Table 6.1 *The Thatcher reforms and beyond*

Post-1990 Trust providers	Position by 2000
Freedom to set pay and conditions locally – not exercised widely	This freedom was removed by the incoming Labour Government
Light touch performance management, separate from the main NHS	Performance management had reverted to regional health authorities and after 1997 central government reasserted even more control
Assets transferred to the Trust	No change
Ability to draw up contracts	Retained but with limits on capital
Limited freedom to make capital decisions	Capital rationing and approval taken back centrally but some capital freedoms retained
Board of executive and non-executive directors with full budgetary responsibility	No change but de facto CEOs became subject to appointment and removal by higher tiers, as well as their board
Senior medical staff employed by the Trust rather than regional authorities	No change
Purchaser–provider split introduced	Retained, but weakened
Ability to retain surpluses	Eroded – required to break even each year; this was then extended to being able to break even over a three-year period, provided certain centrally set conditions were met
Autonomy granted and could be withdrawn if performance was poor	Autonomy was expected to be earned in return for improved performance

6.2.2 Change under Labour, 2001–2010

The 2000 NHS Plan contains a number of important proposals, but most of these were to be driven by central initiatives. By 2002 it was becoming clear that the Department of Health's highly centralized performance management regime was creating significant collateral damage. It centralized blame and forced politicians to become involved in the minutiae of hospital management, reaching its nadir when the Secretary of State found himself explaining in detail why bodies had been left on the floor of the chapel of rest at Bedford Hospital (Bosanquet, 2008). There was also concern that the regime was increasingly felt to be destroying initiative and alienating clinical staff.

The Secretary of State and his advisors looked for alternative approaches to creating radical reform in the NHS, including self-governing organizations and the greater use of incentives and quasi-market mechanisms – although in fact many of the trappings of central performance management remained in place. Following visits to autonomous hospitals in Spain and Sweden, the Secretary of State announced that hospitals that met certain performance criteria would be allowed to apply to become NHS Foundation Trusts. The Labour Government promoted this reform but the model was in fact copied from approaches that were modified versions of the original Thatcher reforms. The publication of an updated NHS Plan containing these proposals was part of a wider package of changes to the reform process, which introduced more reliance on incentives and quasi-market mechanisms. This can be seen as part of a long-term direction in which the NHS has moved from being a monolithic organization to becoming a more loosely connected system and eventually (after 2010) a more regulated industry (Department of Health, 2002).

New governance model

Foundation Trusts were announced as a new governance model, with some important new characteristics enshrined in the Health and Social Care (Community Health and Standards) Act 2003 (HM Government, 2003).

- They were established as public benefit corporations, a novel form of organization with a legal status specifically designed for the purpose of creating Foundation Trusts.

- They had a new form of governance designed to create greater connection with and accountability to local people, patients and staff, who could become members of the Foundation Trusts. Foundation Trust members could form a constituency to which the organization would be accountable and could elect governors responsible for appointing board members.

- Foundation Trusts were allowed to tailor their governance arrangements for local circumstances, in contrast to the heavily prescribed model in the rest of the NHS. While each constitution was unique to the NHS Foundation Trust to which it related, legal requirements were set for the governance structure that applies to all NHS Foundation Trusts.

- Foundation Trusts were to be allowed to retain surpluses.

- They could borrow commercially (within a defined code) and invest in capital. They had access to public capital but PFI deals (a procurement method for the NHS and other parts of the public sector) had to be underwritten by the Secretary of State.

- They could set up joint ventures and other subsidiary businesses.

- Foundation Trusts could sell surplus land and buildings but assets were "locked" to prevent privatization of the provision of health care.

- To change the culture of the organization and make it more innovative, entrepreneurial and responsive to its different constituencies, Foundation Trusts were granted freedom from direct instruction by the Secretary of State for Health and from top-down performance management by the regional tier of the NHS.

- The legislation stipulated that a failure procedure would be designed, which would differ from the commercial insolvency scheme applied to normal enterprises. This was necessary because the assets of the Foundation Trust are "locked" and they cannot be used to guarantee debt or sold to pay creditors. However, developing this regime based on commercial principles proved to be very difficult and after four years it was decided that in case of failure the Foundation Trust would be de-authorized and returned to the management of the Secretary of State for Health.

The role of overseeing financial stability and compliance with regulatory standards was split: a regulator for Foundation Trusts (known as Monitor) was made responsible for ensuring financial viability and compliance with the terms of the Foundation Trust's licence, and the Healthcare Commission (now the Care Quality Commission) became responsible for ensuring compliance with regulatory standards for quality and safety for all public and private providers. The proposal to create Foundation Trusts was politically controversial, both with trade unions and some members of parliament. They were concerned that the measure threatened to reduce accountability and could undermine centrally negotiated pay and conditions – a key source of power and influence for the unions. There was also some concern that the hospitals would pursue private patient income and that the profit motive would undermine NHS values.

As a concession, it was agreed to limit the percentage of private patient income that a Foundation Trust was able to earn to the level it was at when the organization was an NHS Trust in 2002–2003. However, this has proved to be counter-productive as it has prevented some organizations – from which the private patient portion of their income has grown – from becoming Foundation Trusts.

Foundation Trusts were required to sign up to national terms and conditions for staff, although they had some freedoms in this area, examined in more detail in subsection 6.6.3. The proposal to allow borrowing freedoms was resisted by HM Treasury (the United Kingdom's economics and finance ministry) as it removed an important lever to control public sector borrowing and capital

---

Box 6.2 *University College London Hospitals NHS Foundation Trust*[1]

The hospitals which make up University College London Hospitals (UCLH) are:

> University College Hospital
> Eastman Dental Hospital
> Hospital for Tropical Diseases
> National Hospital for Neurology and Neurosurgery
> The Heart Hospital
> The Royal London Homoeopathic Hospital.

The organization has a turnover of €770 million and contracts with over 150 Primary Care Trusts to provide services. The Trust provides more than 500 000 outpatient appointments and more than 100 000 inpatient and day-case admissions each year.

It is a major research centre and has funding from the Government's National Institute for Health Research, for its Biomedical Research Centre. Income to support research infrastructure is over €60 million. In partnership with UCL, the Trust has recently been designated as an Academic Health Sciences Centre, modelled on similar partnerships in the United States.[2]

UCLH has close links with the Royal Free and University College Medical School and London South Bank and City universities to offer training and education for the doctors, nurses, midwives and associated health care professionals.

UCLH became a Foundation Trust in 2004, the first year of the policy's operation.

The Trust is proud of its high-quality outcomes. It has developed a strategy of actively recruiting high-quality academic clinicians, assisted by its close association with one of the top universities in Europe.

---

1 For more details, see the UCLH Foundation Trust web site (http://www.uclh.nhs.uk/Pages/home.aspx, accessed 10 July 2011).
2 For a history of this, see Blumenthal & Edwards (2000).

expenditure; for national accounts, Foundation Trust borrowing counts against the overall public borrowing requirement. After some high-profile political negotiation, it was agreed that Foundation Trust borrowing would remain part of the capital expenditure limit of the Department of Health and that the new regulator, Monitor, would design a prudential borrowing regime. A fourth, less-political concern related to the experience of the quasi-market operating in the 1990s, in which organizations sometimes failed to cooperate appropriately within the wider system. A significant amount of United Kingdom government policy requires cross-organizational working, so Foundation Trusts became obliged to cooperate with other parts of the health system.

Initially it was envisaged that Foundation Trust status would not necessarily be universal. However, in common with previous policy designed to create an "elite" form of organization, it quickly became clear that the Department of Health expected Foundation Trust status to become the default position and that organizations would be required to achieve Foundation Trust status relatively quickly.

6.3 Foundation Trust status

NHS providers of hospital, mental health and ambulance services can apply to be a Foundation Trust when they are capable of demonstrating that they meet the performance, governance and other criteria.

6.3.1 The application process

Applicant organizations must complete a three-part process.

Strategic Health Authority-led trust development phase

The purpose of the development phase[12] is to prepare NHS Trusts for the application process and Secretary of State support; this consists of the preparation of a draft business plan and financial model, a 12-week public consultation on the proposal and a final assessment of the business plan. Entry into the application process is controlled by the regional strategic health authorities (SHAs) and they were often reluctant to initiate the process in circumstances in which they have not determined the strategy for shaping the local health care system. The former executive chair of Monitor also raised questions regarding the SHAs' capability to undertake the development of new Foundation Trusts and their interest in the process (Health Policy Insight, 2010). As a consequence of this and because of the

---

12 Monitor, 2010b.

effect of the economic downturn on Trusts' financial plans, the Department of Health's target for organizations achieving Foundation Trust status has been revised so that all organizations must have become a Foundation Trust, or part of a Foundation Trust through take-over, by April 2013.

The SHA reviews the application against seven criteria, as detailed here. The SHA checks that:

- the organization is legally constituted and has carried out the consultation with the public as required by the legislation; they must also demonstrate that they have a sufficiently large and representative membership to allow them to conduct elections for governors (see subsection 6.7.3 for an explanation of these groups);

- there is a viable business strategy that is consistent with the strategy of their purchasers on which consultations have been carried out;

- the organization is financially viable and has well-developed approaches to long-term financial planning;

- the quality of its existing governance arrangements is sufficiently high, including risk management, compliance with regulatory standards, evidence of ability to meet statutory targets, and performance management systems;

- the individuals that make up the board are fully capable, especially to deal with any potential conflicts of interest that may arise; and

- the organization's record of performance is suitable, including relating to the delivery of government targets, such as waiting times in the emergency room, and waiting time targets for planned surgery; the characteristics of the local health system are also assessed to ensure the financial performance of purchasers does not pose a threat and to check that other strategic changes (such as plans to change services) will not destabilize the organization.

Secretary of State support phase

Having passed the first phase of assurance, the Trust can then seek the approval of the Secretary of State. The SHA has to demonstrate that the applicant Trust is fit for purpose to a committee convened by the Department of Health.

Monitor phase

In this phase, Monitor assesses whether the Trust meets the standard required. Three criteria are used to assess this: (1) Is the Trust well governed? (2) Is it financially viable? (3) Is it legally constituted? Organizations that have been subject to review by Monitor report that it is a very robust and rigorous process and often significantly more challenging than previous NHS organizational or performance reviews. Monitor has been very clear that it is not willing to lower its entry criteria to meet a political timetable for organizations to achieve Foundation Trust status.

6.3.2 The conditions for becoming a Foundation Trust

When Foundation Trusts are authorized, the terms of their licence specifies the broad range of services that they are required to provide in order to ensure they are meeting their obligations as part of a public health care system. The licence includes:

- a description of the health services that an NHS Foundation Trust is authorized to provide;

- a list of services that the Foundation Trust is required to provide to the NHS in England – this may include teaching and research functions as well as health services;

- a requirement to operate according to national standards and targets;

- the circumstances in which major changes to services (for example, in response to a changing local population) need to be discussed locally and agreed by Monitor;

- a list of assets, such as buildings, land or equipment, that are designated as "protected" because they are needed to provide required NHS services;

- the amount of money an NHS Foundation Trust is allowed to borrow;

- the financial and statistical information an NHS Foundation Trust is required to provide; and

- the private patient income limit.

The rationale for specifying services that the Foundation Trust is required to provide is that organizations might choose to stop providing loss-making essential services in favour of more profitable activity. The United Kingdom's relatively concentrated pattern of hospital provision means that many hospitals enjoy a monopoly position for a number of services, in particular in emergency care, and so the unplanned exit of a provider would present a problem in many areas.

6.3.3 Deauthorization

Foundation Trust status can be withdrawn through a de-authorization process. Monitor has the power to do this if the terms of the licence have been breached in a sufficiently serious way and remedial action is either inappropriate because of the scale of the problem or has failed. However, Monitor must consult the regional SHA and the payers involved.

The grounds for de-authorization were extended in the 2009 Health Act and include action where there is serious concern regarding:

- the health and safety of patients

- the quality of the provision by the Trust of goods and services

- the financial position of the Trust

- the way the Trust is being run.

If de-authorized, the Trust is returned to the control of the Secretary of State. If it has not already been removed, the Secretary of State can replace the Board and has powers to appoint an administrator to produce proposals for the future of the organization, including options for closure, breaking it up or having it taken over. To date, these powers have not been used and are expected to be only employed in the most extreme circumstances.

In what was seen by some as an attempt to reassert some form of political control over Foundation Trusts, the 2009 Act contains a power to ask Monitor to consider de-authorization if the Secretary of State considers that there has been a serious enough breach of its licence. It would be difficult for Monitor to resist such a request, but it can refuse de-authorization provided it can justify its reasons. Many commentators thought this represented some reassertion of central authority in an otherwise politically "arm's-length" process.

6.4 Strategic governance

Foundation Trusts are embedded in wider health care systems and so their objectives are obviously shaped accordingly. The NHS has become increasingly diverse in recent years, leading to more interest in the shared principles and values that hold it together. As part of this, organizations are now expected to follow a set of principles for cooperation and competition, overseen by an advisory panel appointed by government. More recently, an NHS Constitution was developed to articulate the underlying values of the NHS as a whole and define what is offered to patients and staff (Department of Health, 2010c).

6.4.1 The shape of services

Creating Foundation Trusts changed the governance of organizations, rather than their configuration. In common with most hospitals becoming

Foundation Trusts, UCLH determined the shape of its organization some time before applying for Foundation Trust status. The NHS has seen a significant number of mergers between hospitals since the early 1990s, driven by the need to reconfigure clinical services and in some cases the potential for economies of scope and scale. Comparable to what happened at UCLH, provider organizations that are now becoming Foundation Trusts are inheriting this legacy.

It is likely that organizations not in a position to become Foundation Trusts by 2015 will be taken over or split up. However, the process for this is not yet clear and, while central government and regional authorities are keen to see Foundation Trusts take over struggling organizations, there are few incentives to do so, especially given that hospital mergers have historically been very disappointing in terms of their general failure to achieve their proposed goals.

Instead, there is significantly more interest in various types of "vertical integration", including the management of services outside of hospitals, and partnerships with primary care. UCLH is considering options for developing more outpatient services closely related to some of its own specialist services. In common with a number of other hospitals, UCLH is also interested in the potential to become sufficiently integrated to receive a capitation payment for care for a defined population group, but this would require some changes in the current policy framework.

6.5 Financial management

6.5.1 Financial freedoms

Foundation Trusts have significant financial freedoms, including procurement, how they invest spare cash, and setting their annual budget. But the principles of probity and transparency in the use of public money, which apply to all government bodies, also apply to Foundation Trusts (HM Treasury, 2009). Monitor's risk-rating process determines the extent to which the organization may borrow funds.

Foundation Trust boards have complete freedom to choose their level of surplus (in the case of UCLH this is about 2.7% of income before exceptional items), although this is an important point of debate with the governors, who would prefer to have a lower surplus and more money to be dedicated to improving quality and service to patients. The level of contingency reserves, procurement decisions and the target for the risk rating assessed by Monitor are all within the full discretion of the Trust.

6.5.2 Mergers, acquisitions and investments

Mergers with other organizations require the Foundation Trust to be dissolved and reconstituted using Monitor's assessment process, which is used to assess the initial application. This – along with the appropriate due diligence investigation – makes the process potentially expensive and time consuming. UCLH regards the merger process as unwieldy and the requirement to dissolve the existing organizations as a complete barrier to its use as a method of expansion. By comparison, acquisitions – while still requiring significant investment in time – appear to be a much more accessible route to organizational change. There have been four major acquisitions at UCLH since the start of the Foundation Trust process, three in mental health services and one in general hospital services.

Acquisitions, investments and high-risk transactions – for example, involving equity, securities, profit shares, royalties – must be reported to Monitor, which has issued guidance designed to encourage a prudent approach. Yet this only applies to funds generated by activities for the NHS and not to any charitable funds owned by the Trust. This represents an important shift from a situation in which mergers were often promoted by regional SHAs, sometimes against the wishes of local organizations. It also makes the decision-making process for mergers and investment much more rigorous than previously, and has significantly weakened the role of external bodies such as the regional SHA.

Foundation Trusts have freedom to borrow within the prudential borrowing scheme set by Monitor. They also have access to low-cost finance from the Foundation Trust Financing Facility, a Department of Health internal banking function that treats applications on a commercial basis. However, Trusts that have used this report that the facility has been difficult to access and somewhat risk averse. Foundation Trusts may also enter into private patient partnership and PFI deals, although these may require underwriting by the Secretary of State, who remains the residual owner in cases of insolvency.

UCLH recently decided to invest £100 million in a new cancer centre, funded through a combination of land and property sales and a loan from the Foundation Trust Financing Facility. Obviously the views of payers, the university, the regional SHA and other bodies with an interest were taken into account, but the board has the authority to make the final decision. In this case, Monitor was consulted but its role was to ensure compliance with the regulatory procedure relating to borrowing, not to review the decision itself.

6.5.3 Joint ventures and commercial undertakings

Foundation Trusts are allowed to form joint ventures and run commercial businesses, provided this is in line with their (generally permissive) licence.

However, a recent court decision has inhibited this: a case brought by a trade union found that income from joint ventures that provide non-NHS health care must be counted as part of the Foundation Trust's private patient income.

UCLH has a number of commercial activities, including the outsourcing of its private medical services to a specialist company.

6.6 Operational governance

6.6.1 Management structures

All Foundation Trusts have complete discretion in the design of their management structures.

UCLH has opted for a divisional structure with four divisions headed by a medical director (usually, but not exclusively, a doctor) supported by management and accounting staff. These divisions have full income and expenditure responsibility and recharging is possible for the use of common services. However, managing profit and loss is not delegated, as decisions on cross-subsidization must be made centrally, to avoid some perverse incentives and to ensure the optimal use of shared facilities, such as laboratories. Decisions to procure these from outside of the Trust could damage important services and leave fixed costs uncovered. At UCLH, the four divisions operate with their own Boards of Management and are held to account for the delivery of performance targets, financial performance, and quality and safety standards. Overseeing quality and safety, external reporting and the identification of emerging trends not identifiable at directorate level is the responsibility of a central team.

The managers of the four divisions have a high level of discretion within the parameters set by the Trust Board and the Trust's annual business plan.

6.6.2 Performance management

Foundation Trusts are subject to a large number of externally set performance requirements from a number of sources:

* government targets and standards for speed of treatment in the emergency room; maximum referral to treatment times; waiting times for cancer treatment; health care-associated infections, and so on;

* performance requirements and quality standards set by payers, including a small element of pay-for-performance contracting;

* regulatory requirements set by the Care Quality Commission (see subsection 6.7.5); and

- Monitor's financial risk and governance requirements.

These last two relate more to achieving minimum standards, and the government has pledged not to introduce new targets. Within this relatively prescriptive framework, the Trust can set its own performance management targets.

UCLH has a very sophisticated internal performance management system, which provides the Management Board, clinical boards and managers with detailed information. It is designed based on the organization's top-10 priorities, including a number of externally set requirements, but most are set through an iterative process within the organization, and sub-objectives are set for most of these. The requirements for individual managers and departments are derived from these corporate priorities and are incorporated into the appraisal requirements for individuals. The priorities and sub-objectives are reviewed frequently (at least once a quarter) with individual directorates being asked to present to the UCLH Board on their progress.

6.6.3 Human resources and workforce

Foundation Trusts are free to determine numbers of staff they need and to hire and fire. When they were established, they were required to accept the nationally negotiated pay system and existing staff have a contractual right to the terms of the national contract and pay systems. Foundation Trusts can only alter terms by agreement, or by terminating and reissuing new contracts, which is a legal minefield in United Kingdom law. For new staff, Foundation Trusts could choose to pay their own rates, but this would create some risk of challenge on equal pay grounds. A small number of Foundation Trusts have created new roles, for example support worker roles or physicians' assistants. If used properly, there is also considerable scope for this within the national pay arrangements. One Trust has its own full-fledged pay structure and a few have more limited organizational bonus schemes. A sizeable number have changed managerial pay arrangements. It is likely that over time there will be much more interest in moving to more localized pay arrangements.

Pay

The history of a nationally negotiated deal for pay, conditions and contracts of employment means that the expertise and infrastructure for this has not been developed in individual organizations. The costs of developing this are thought to be high and there is risk associated with being an early innovator or first mover, as staff might leave for other organizations with more advantageous terms.

There are also some political hazards. The trade unions have a strong interest in preserving national negotiation. It is anticipated that over time there will be some further moves for Foundation Trusts to negotiate significant variations from national pay and conditions; this may need to be carried out in regional groups. At present, UCLH has no plans to depart from nationally set pay and conditions.

6.7 Accountability framework

Foundation Trust boards are responsible for the management of the hospital and a Board of Governors – elected from a constituency consisting of the members of the Foundation Trust and a number of appointed governors – appoint board members. External scrutiny is exercised by Monitor, purchasers, local government and a number of external regulators. Each of these elements is examined below.

6.7 1 The Board

The Board is responsible for the overall governance of the Foundation Trust, its strategy, compliance with regulatory requirements and overall performance. The chair and non-executive directors are appointed by the governors, who also approve the choice of CEO made by the Board. The Board must have a CEO and a finance director, and the Act specifies that there should be a medical practitioner and a nurse among the executive directors (HM Government, 2006). There is a requirement for there to be a majority or equal number of non-executives. Beyond this, there is considerable freedom regarding how the Board is constituted, how often it meets, whether it meets in public and how business is conducted. See Box 6.3 for more detail regarding the UCLH Board.

UCLH has taken responsibility for selecting its own non-executive directors and has taken considerable care to ensure that the skills, knowledge and experience of these individuals are complementary to those of other board members. This approach puts the selection of board members beyond the influence of national or local politicians, although clearly there are advantages to appointing individuals who are well connected in terms of political networks and have local influence.

Operational issues, such as performance, financial reporting, quality and other matters relating to the running of the organization dominate discussion at the UCLH Board, but the Trust estimates that about 30% of the Board's time is dedicated to long-term and strategic issues. A small Executive Board meets weekly, with one meeting a month involving a wider group of senior leaders – this tends to focus on some aspect of change management or planning.

Box 6.3 *The UCLH Board*

Board members

> Chairman
>
> CEO
>
> Deputy chief executive
>
> Chief nurse
>
> Medical director
>
> Finance director
>
> Workforce director
>
> Non-executive directors x 5.

What is the role of the Board?

- To set the overall policy and strategic direction for the Trust.
- To approve and monitor UCLHs' business plans, budgets and major capital expenditure.
- To monitor performance against objectives.
- To be members of committees such as the remuneration committee and audit committee.

What are the responsibilities of the Board?

- As the board of a public service body, the Board should meet regularly, retain full and effective control over the organization and monitor the executive management of the Trust.
- Board members have corporate responsibility for:
  - establishing the strategic direction of UCLH within the policy and funding framework set out by parliament;
  - defining annual and longer-term objectives and agreeing plans to achieve them;
  - overseeing the delivery of planned results by monitoring performance against agreed objectives and targets, ensuring corrective action is taken when necessary;
  - establishing an effective system of corporate governance;
  - safeguarding the public reputation of the Trust; and
  - supporting internal and external communications and participating in meetings with other external organizations.

Source: UCLH, 2011a.

6.7.2 Members

The rhetoric underpinning the creation of Foundation Trusts was largely about autonomy to free decisions from central government interference. The concept of a transfer of ownership was also significant in discussions and reference was made to the tradition of mutual organizations when the original policy was discussed. The idea that the Trust would be owned by its members was thought to have significant advantages in changing the orientation of the organization to a more focused approach to the needs of its users, rather than those of government. It was also thought that this would increase the stake that staff, patients and the public had in the organization and would bring significant and more diverse influences to bear on the development of its strategy. Originally, it was proposed that members should pay £1 in equity – forfeit if the organization was wound up – to create a sense of ownership, but this idea was dropped, as the costs associated with it were high and the gesture largely symbolic.

Trusts applying for Foundation Trust status are required to demonstrate a robust strategy for engaging people as members and to ensure that they match the socioeconomic, ethnic and other characteristics of their patients, local public and staff. Where appropriate, children and young people are also encouraged to join. In March 2010, the 129 Foundation Trusts had about 1.6 million members between them.

6.7.3 Governors

Typically, Foundation Trusts have between 18 and 39 governors, with an average of 33 (see Box 6.4). The size and composition of their Board of Governors is determined locally but the legislation specifies that every Board of Governors must have:

- a majority of governors elected by members within the public constituency;

- at least one governor representing local NHS PCTs;

- at least one governor representing local (government) authorities in the area;

- at least three governors representing staff; and

- at least one governor appointed from the local university (if the trust's hospitals include a medical or dental school).

Governors are required to meet three times a year, although in a review of Foundation Trust membership, Ham and Hunt (2008) found that governors tend to meet more frequently than this (Ham & Hunt, 2008). There is obviously some risk of overlap with the responsibilities of the Executive Board, but three key roles are identified for governors. First, they form an advisory body that provides a viewpoint on how the Foundation Trust should operate to meet the needs of the members of the wider community. Second, they act as guardians to ensure that the Trust operates in a way that fits its statement of purpose and complies with the terms of its authorization. Third, governors have a strategic role advising on the longer term direction of the Foundation Trust.

Box 6.4 *UCLH governors and members*

The governing body is composed of 33 people, 23 of whom are elected by the Trust's patient, public and staff members. A total of 3 governors represent the local public, 14 represent patients and 6 represent staff; 10 other governors are appointed by local partner organizations, including the PCT and university. Elections to the governing body are held each year.

Members are drawn from among local people, recent patients, their carers and staff. In April 2009, the Trust had 14 000 members.

There are three formal meetings a year, a joint meeting with the Board and an Annual General Meeting. There are also a number of informal meetings and subcommittees dealing with various matters, including remuneration, patient issues and high-quality patient care. Governors also sit on the subcommittees of the Trust.

Communication between governors and their constituencies is managed by the Trust through regular newsletters and the organization of informal meetings.

Source: UCLH, 2011b.

It is not yet clear to what extent governors exert real influence over the operation of Foundation Trusts. Meeting minutes suggest that a significant amount of the business consists of executives reporting on recent developments and explaining the context in which the organization is operating. There is much less evidence of active challenge by the governors or of them setting a significant amount of the organization's agenda. However, it is clear that UCLH Governors have played an important role, particularly in terms of quality and safety issues and matters relating to patients. The system is in the early stages of development and it would be premature to make any judgement regarding how effective this model is likely to be. Research into governors' opinions in 2008 found that they had a good understanding of their role, were generally satisfied with the level of involvement they had with their Trusts' executives and felt that they understood the organization's strategy. Their role in representing the community was thought to be important, although they reported that ensuring that they were really being representative was challenging (Ipsos MORI, 2008). More recent research suggests that, while governors have the potential to exert significant influence through their power to appoint the Board, this has not been realized. They often felt that they were easily controlled by CEOs and did not have access to information to allow them to exercise their role. The researchers comment, "governors reported that they did not feel that directors genuinely expected them to make any significant input" (Dixon, Storey & Rosete, 2010).

Research conducted in 2005 found that many of the elections for governors were competitive and there was more than one candidate for 85% of the posts of governor appointed from among the public and 73% of the posts of governor appointed from among patients (Lewis, 2005). However, the turnout rate varied between NHS Foundation Trusts, from 19% to 67% for the posts of governor taken from the public, and 31% to 70% for patient governors. Initially average turnout reached 40%, but the most recent data suggest that the figure has fallen to 27%, with 20% of governor positions being uncontested. Turnout for staff governors was the lowest and in 37% of cases there was only one candidate (House of Commons, 2009).

6.7.4 Monitor

Monitor, the regulator of Foundation Trusts, is responsible for authorizing new Foundation Trusts, as well as playing an active role in developing organizational capability within all Foundation Trusts. Monitor is independent of government and responsible directly to Parliament (Monitor, 2010c). Its regulatory role is to ensure that Foundation Trusts comply with their terms of authorization, including:

• the requirement to operate effectively, efficiently and economically

• requirements to meet health care targets and national standards

• the requirement to cooperate with other NHS organizations.

Monitor regards the Board as the first line of regulation in NHS Foundation Trusts. It receives an annual plan and regular reports on performance and uses these to exercise its judgement on organizational matters and to identify where problems might arise. This includes calculating an annual risk rating, from an annual plan with financial projections, which gives an assessment of the probability that the Trust will breach the terms of its authorization. The rating then determines how closely Monitor will examine the Trust's performance. Monitor (2010a, p. 5) states that "a successful NHS Foundation Trust can expect to be given considerable latitude to exercise its freedoms. Financially secure NHS Foundation Trusts are given an increased ability to borrow. Monitor will not involve itself in determining health care strategy or operational policies in NHS Foundation Trusts." This risk-based approach has been consistently applied and is well received by Foundation Trusts. Within these constraints there is a very high degree of freedom.

Monitor reviews risk ratings relating to financial performance and governance on a quarterly basis. This includes the organization's performance in the delivery of national targets: for example, waiting times in accident and emergency departments, infection rates, and so on. On occasions, Monitor has also shown itself to be concerned about decisions made by boards which appear to have high levels of risk associated with them. Monitor has intervention powers where Foundation Trusts have high levels of risk or are in significant breach of their terms of authorization.

Initially, Monitor did not concern itself with issues relating to quality, other than in areas that were government targets for improvement or compliance. However, a number of well-publicized problems in some hospitals, one of which was a Foundation Trust, has led to the regulator taking a more active role in ensuring that Foundation Trusts have systems for ensuring high performance in managing infections, quality and safety. Even so, it has been selective and targeted in taking a risk-based approach, tending to favour approaches to encourage problem solving and improvement, for example, with organizations failing in their performance on national targets relating to methicillin-resistant *Staphylococcus aureus* (MRSA) bacteraemias or thrombolysis in myocardial infarction.

Although it is a well-managed and successful organization, UCLH has had some experience of Monitor's intervention procedure. For a period it experienced a serious financial problem resulting from an increased need for funds in order to pay the initial charge for the new PFI hospital, which – had the organization not become a Foundation Trust – would have been underwritten by the Department of Health. This resulted in Monitor exercising its intervention powers to require the appointment of a financial turnaround team to work alongside the Trust's management. Once a sound financial regime had been restored, the relationship reverted to being at arm's length.

That the Board was not removed is unusual in such a case, and reflected the fact that the problem was outside the control of the Trust. In circumstances in which there has been a loss of financial control or other serious breaches of governance, the Board (or substantial parts of it) have been replaced by direct action by Monitor.

Monitor has shown itself to be a very sophisticated regulator, with the ability to make accurate judgements regarding the level of risk to which Foundation Trusts are exposed in terms of their business strategy and finances. This has been extended in recent years to paying more attention to the quality of services.

In addition to the functions of authorizing and regulating Foundation Trusts, the third strand of Monitor's work is focused on supporting their development to ensure they take full advantage of the freedoms that accompany Foundation Trust status.

The level of supervision that Monitor exercises is based on its perception of risk, which has limited the burden of regulation on hospitals. It has also assisted in the attempt to change the culture of continually looking upward for direction.

It has taken some time for previously directly supervised hospitals to learn a new more independent form of operation, and Monitor has commented that Trusts are still too ready to refer questions to them that are actually within their own competence to decide. This is changing. Senior UCLH staff report that Monitor is viewed as an important body and that its opinion is influential. It is seen as being helpful in providing advice and has been very careful to stay within its mandate and avoid interfering in wider operational and strategic issues.

6.7.5 Other external scrutiny

The main external regulator is the Care Quality Commission (previously the Healthcare Commission), which sets minimum standards and legally registers all organizations that provide NHS services. All providers are required to satisfy the regulator that they meet a range of minimum standards, and internal assurance processes are in place to ensure that they continue to do so. Some of this is carried out via self-assessment against published standards, supplemented by analysis of data and periodic and unannounced inspections.

All hospitals – Foundation Trusts or otherwise – are answerable to a number of other external regulatory bodies, which all require information to be reported.

These include:

- the Health and Safety Executive
- the Clinical Negligence Scheme – a mutual insurance scheme
- regulators for fertility treatment and tissues
- local fire and environmental health authorities
- bodies responsible for approving postgraduate medical education and training.

In common with other NHS organizations, Foundation Trusts are also subject to external scrutiny by local government oversight committees. These vary significantly in their effectiveness and capacities; their direct powers are limited, although they have the statutory right to be consulted. However, they have the power to object to large-scale changes and refer these objections to the Secretary of State (who can only intervene if the Foundation Trust is in breach of its licence).

6.7.6 Payers

In a significant number of cases a Foundation Trust will have one PCT that is the majority purchaser of its services. This gives them potentially a great deal of influence, but also means there are limits relating to how far they can take action that threatens the survival of the organization. PCTs have become active in trying to influence the shape of patient pathways and the location of certain specialist activities. UCLH has no single PCT which has a decisive influence and, unusually, the two PCTs covering the local population only represent 19% of total income.

6.7.7 Reporting to the public

There is an increasing expectation that public bodies are transparently held to account for the quality of their services and their use of public money. Each Foundation Trust is required to produce an annual report covering the activities of the Trust, its performance against its objectives and information for local people and patients regarding how it is performing. This must include a full set of financial accounts, with information on the remuneration of the senior executives and, since 2010, a quality account (see Box 6.5).

Box 6.5 *UCLH quality account*

UCLH has been piloting the development of quality accounts. These include some nationally mandated information, but the Trust has chosen to focus on five areas:

1. to achieve an overall patient satisfaction rating in the top 20 NHS hospitals;
2. to achieve a reduction in the hospital mortality rate of 5%;
3. to reduce the incidence of all falls, and those with serious injury, by at least 30%;
4. to reduce the level of health care associated infections; and
5. continuous quality improvement – to develop quality "dashboards"[1] in all divisions in the coming year, with indicators and goals relating to patient experience, safety and effective treatment with good outcomes.

The account contains:

1. the Trusts' performance in the view of regulators and Monitor;
2. responses to feedback from public engagement activities; and
3. performance on a wide range of quality measures, including:
   - safety
   - infections
   - mortality rates
   - patient experience
   - patient outcomes
   - staff views
   - performance against key external targets.

---

1 A set of aggregated indicators designed to measure the performance of the organization.

Foundation Trusts are subject to the same requirements as all public sector organizations in terms of disclosure under freedom of information legislation. There is a legal requirement for substantial changes to be subject to extensive public consultation. Generally speaking, this responsibility is exercised by purchasers, but in certain circumstances the Foundation Trust would be required to do this – for example, in the event that it is instigating a major change in services or in the location(s) at which they are provided.

The UCLH Board meets in public, although there is no requirement to do so, and a significant number of Foundation Trust Boards meet in private, despite some exhortation from ministers that they should not. Boards can meet in closed session when they need to deal with commercially sensitive issues or where patient confidentiality may be an issue. The remuneration committee report is carried out in the public part of the UCLH Board meeting and the pay of senior managers is reported in the Annual Report. The governors meet in public.

6.8 Changes since May 2010

Following the general election in May 2010, the new coalition government has announced a programme of very significant changes to the NHS in England – a number of which have important implications for Foundation Trusts (Department of Health, 2010a,b). These include the following measures.

- Trusts will be given freedom to change elements of their constitution with the approval of their Board.

- Some of the barriers to merger will be removed – particularly the requirement to dissolve the boards of merging organizations.

- Barriers to organizations taking over others will also be reduced, although the effect of this may be somewhat offset by the introduction of a new and powerful regulator to enforce competition policy.

- For some providers, the possibility of having a staff-only membership will be considered.

- Restrictions on Foundation Trusts' ability to earn income from private medicine and other sources will be removed.

- The potential to remove the restrictions imposed on Foundation Trust borrowing will be considered. This is to be accompanied by removing access to government capital for major investment programmes.

- Monitor's role in overseeing Foundation Trusts' performance and compliance with the terms of their authorization or other aspects of performance management will be removed. This is a very significant change, as it removes the oversight of the management of Foundation Trusts and is a further step towards much greater autonomy. While Monitor will remain as a regulatory organization, it will take responsibility for price setting, the economic regulation of the health care market, competition regulation and setting licensing conditions for the provision of essential local services – that is, where continuity is required and there is a need to ensure that providers cannot withdraw services without notice.

- To reflect these changes and as an additional safeguard for the assets for which the state remains the owner, as well as to redress perceived shortcomings in accountability, the government will consider whether to strengthen the nature of the accountability to the organization's governors by giving them additional powers. The forthcoming Health and Social Care Bill will make explicit the duty of governors to hold the Board of Directors to account, through the chair and non-executive directors (whom they have power to appoint and remove). It will also give governors power to require some or all of the Trust's directors to attend a meeting. For transparency, the Foundation Trust's annual report would have to list any occasions on which this power was used. It will extend to Foundation Trust directors the duties imposed on directors under company law, such as the requirement to promote the success of the organization.

- Foundation Trusts will be required to hold an annual general meeting for its membership, at which members would be able to discuss the Trust's annual report and accounts, including the remuneration of directors.

The regime in which the Foundation Trusts operate will move to being one based more on the rules of a market. This will include the adoption of an approach to insolvency based on commercial law and may lead to the removal of some competitive advantages accruing to Foundation Trusts, gained when they were under state control. These include the state underwriting of a generous pension scheme, access to borrowing at advantageous rates, access to trainee staff and some tax advantages. In addition, the government intends to remove a large number of the performance targets that have been used to create pressure for performance improvement in the system.

If all of these changes are enacted, the impact on Foundation Trusts will be very significant. In particular, the level of oversight provided by external organizations will be greatly reduced. Foundation Trusts will be much more "on their own" and will take complete responsibility for ensuring that they are successful.

At the same time, a much more pluralistic and potentially competitive market for providers will be established and there will be changes in responsibility for purchasing that may make the environment more dynamic.

There are a number of unresolved issues. Liabilities and commitments as part of the PFI are currently underwritten by the state and are a barrier to more flexible models of care delivery. The state retains substantial interests (in the form of debt) in the Foundation Trusts and this is an obstacle to the development of a private banking market to support Foundation Trusts in making changes.

6.9 Success and sustainability of the model

Reaching a consensus on the success of the model is difficult because of the significant level of policy (and other) change since the mid-1990s and the fact that the criteria for becoming a Foundation Trust meant that early applicants were already successful organizations. A further problem is that for much of the period, policy was directed at improving providers; the purchasing function was left undeveloped and subjected to a very disruptive and extensive programme of restructuring.

Monitor's analysis seems to suggest that the process of becoming a Foundation Trust had a significant and beneficial impact on the quality of financial control, strategic planning and governance arrangements. It suggests that, while the sector has started to innovate and change, progress has been significantly less marked than the advocates of the policy predicted and that post-assessment Foundation Trusts did not improve any faster than non-Foundation Trusts (Monitor, 2009). The reasons for this might include the following elements.

- There is a strong cultural legacy persisting since 1948 relating to the way the NHS has been managed as a highly centralized institution, in which the expectation was that new ideas and strategic direction came from the top.

- The underdeveloped purchasing function meant that it was difficult to obtain payer approval for new services.

- Payers and providers still had a very long list of targets and requirements with which to comply, which absorbed managerial time.

- There is relatively limited competitive threat to hospitals, due to the concentrated nature of provision. Early indications from research suggest that increased competition may be more effective than governance changes in improving outcomes and quality.

The example of UCLH seems to suggest that some of these difficulties can be overcome. However, the extent to which UCLH is an indicator for other organizations is questionable, as there are some special factors to consider, including the following: there is a high-quality and stable leadership team in place (including high-calibre clinical leadership); unusually, there is no one payer with a very large share of the hospitals' income; and UCLH has a strong association with a world-class university.

An important question regarding the success of the model is the extent to which it is likely to be sustained in the long term. There was a strong expectation – based on the previous experiment with provider autonomy – that the system would try to reinvent methods to exert control. Indeed, according to the advisor to the Secretary of State at the time at which the policy was being developed, one of the reasons for which the freedoms and governance model were embodied in legislation was to remove politicians' temptation to intervene. It appears that a number of politicians and officials in positions of influence in later years either did not understand or did not support the underlying principles of the policy and have sought to find ways to reassert influence. For example, a very public and somewhat acrimonious debate took place when Monitor objected to the CEO of the NHS writing directly to the CEOs of Foundation Trusts regarding improvements in infection control.

Following a scandal regarding poor care at the Mid Staffordshire Hospital Foundation Trust, the Secretary of State sent in senior officials, despite having no legal power to do so. He was, however, reflecting widespread public and media concern about the apparently unaccountable nature of the Foundation Trust and was responding to an expectation that he would act. This incident led to a widespread questioning of the lack of accountability of the foundation model. The Mid Staffordshire Hospital Foundation Trust appeared to have over-enthusiastically embraced the financial targets required by Monitor and had achieved these by reducing the quality of care, in particular in terms of staffing levels in wards and the emergency department (Francis, 2010). The governance systems failed to identify the deterioration in the quality of services and the regulator, which relies extensively on self-certification, was very slow to identify the problem, as were the purchasers and the regional SHA. They all failed to respond to warning signals, including complaints from an active group of local patients and their carers. This pattern of insular behaviour and a tendency to ignore warning signals has also been found in a number of non-Foundation Trusts and so is not a consequence of the model; rather, it can be seen as giving legitimacy to this pattern of behaviour, where it is already present. The incident was important and led to many commentators questioning whether more intrusive regulation was required. New powers were integrated into legislation to allow the Secretary of State to ask Monitor to consider de-authorization.

The move in the direction of increased independence for providers will now be difficult to reverse, and such increased independence forms an important part of the new government's reform programme.

6.10 References

Blumenthal D, Edwards N (2000). A tale of two systems: the changing academic health center. *Health Affairs*, 19(3):86–101.

Bosanquet N (2008). The health and welfare legacy. In: Seldon A, ed. *Blair's Britain, 1997–2007*. Cambridge, Cambridge University Press:385–407.

Department of Health (2002). *Delivering the NHS plan: next steps on investment, next steps on reform*. London, Department of Health (http://www.dh.gov.uk/en/Publicationsandstatistics/Publications/PublicationsPolicyAndGuidance/DH_4005818, accessed 2 May 2011).

Department of Health (2010a). *Equity and excellence: liberating the NHS*. London, The Stationery Office (Crown Copyright, Cm7881).

Department of Health (2010b.) *Liberating the NHS: legislative framework and next steps*. London, The Stationery Office (Crown Copyright, Cm7993).

Department of Health (2010c). *The NHS Constitution for England (2009 edition)*. London, Department of Health (http://www.dh.gov.uk/en/Publicationsandstatistics/Publications/PublicationsPolicyAndGuidance/DH_113613, accessed 2 May 2011).

Dixon A, Storey J, Rosete AA (2010). Accountability of foundation trusts in the English NHS: views of directors and governors. *Journal of Health Services Research & Policy*, 15(2):82–89.

Francis R (2010). *The mid-Staffordshire NHS foundation trust independent inquiry, January 2005–March 2009*. London, The Stationery Office (http://www.midstaffsinquiry.com/, accessed 2 May 2011) (Crown Copyright, ID 2350504).

Ham C, Hunt P (2008). *Membership governance in NHS foundation trusts: a review for the Department of Health*. London, Department of Health.

Health Policy Insight (2010). Interview – Dr Bill Moyes, Executive Chair, Monitor [web site]. Health Policy Insight (http://www.healthpolicyinsight.com/?q=node/398, accessed December 2010).

HM Government (2003). *Health and Social Care (Community Health and Standards) Act 2003*. London, National Archives (https://www.opsi.gov.uk/acts/acts2003/ukpga_20030043_en_2#pt1-pb4-l1g18, accessed 2 May 2011).

HM Government (2006). *National Health Service Act 2006*. London, National Archives (http://www.opsi.gov.uk/acts/acts2006/ukpga_20060041_en_28#sch7, accessed 2 May 2011).

HM Treasury (2009). Managing public money [web site]. London, HM Treasury (http://www.hm-treasury.gov.uk/psr_mpm_index.htm, accessed 2 May 2011).

House of Commons (2009). *NHS foundation trusts: governing bodies*. Commons Debates (Hansard), Column 1339W, 20 October 2009. London, UK Parliament House of Commons (http://www.publications.parliament.uk/pa/cm200809/cmhansrd/cm091020/text/91020w0005.htm, accessed 2 May 2011).

Ipsos MORI (2008). *Survey of foundation trust governors: research study conducted for Monitor – independent regulator of NHS foundation trusts*. London, Monitor (http://www.monitor-nhsft.gov.uk/sites/default/files/publications/Ipsos_MORI_survey_FT_governors_June2008.pdf, accessed 2 May 2011).

Lewis R (2005). *Governing foundation trusts – a new era for public accountability*. London, The King's Fund.

Monitor (2009). *Measuring Monitor's impact: economic evaluation report*. London, Monitor (http://www.monitor-nhsft.gov.uk/home/our-publications/browse-category/about-monitor/what-we-do/measuring-monitors-impact-economic-ev, accessed 2 May 2011).

Monitor (2010a). *Monitor's compliance philosophy*. London, Monitor (http://www.monitor-nhsft.gov.uk/sites/default/files/publications/part1cf_0.pdf, accessed 14 June 2011).

Monitor (2010b). Phase one – SHA-led trust development phase [web site]. London, Monitor (http://www.monitor-nhsft.gov.uk/home/becoming-nhs-foundation-trust/how-assessment-process-works/phase-one-sha-led-trust-development-, accessed 2 May 2010).

Monitor (2010c). What we do [web site]. London, Monitor (http://www.monitor-nhsft.gov.uk/home/about-monitor/what-we-do, accessed 2 May 2010).

UCLH (2011a). Board of directors [web site]. London, University College London Hospitals NHS Foundation Trust (http://www.uclh.nhs.uk/aboutus/whoweare/bod/Pages/Home.aspx, accessed 2 May 2011).

UCLH (2011b). Governing body [web site]. London, University College London Hospitals NHS Foundation Trust (http://www.uclh.nhs.uk/aboutus/FT/GB/Pages/Home.aspx, accessed 2 May 2011).

Chapter 7
Estonia

Triin Habicht, Jarno Habicht and Maris Jesse

7.1 Introduction: brief overview of the Estonian health care sector

The Estonian health system operates based on compulsory, solidarity-based health insurance and service providers working within the framework of private sector legislation.

Stewardship and supervision – along with health policy development – are the duties of the Ministry of Social Affairs and its agencies.

The financing of health care is a responsibility of the independent Estonian Health Insurance Fund (EHIF), the main role of which is to be an active purchasing agency, and its responsibilities include contracting health care providers and paying for health care services, reimbursing pharmaceutical expenditure and paying for temporary sick leave and maternity benefits. The EHIF is governed by a 15-member Supervisory Board, consisting of representatives from the state, employers and organizations of insured individuals. To ensure consistency between the Ministry of Social Affairs and the EHIF, as well as political accountability, the Supervisory Board is chaired by the Minister of Social Affairs (Habicht, 2008).

Local municipalities have a minor, rather voluntary role in organizing and financing health services. However, most hospitals belong to municipal governments, which either own them outright as limited companies or manage them through non-profit-making "foundations".

Since the passing of the new Health Services Organization Act in May 2001 (with effect from 2002), health care provision has been almost completely decentralized. The Act defines four types of health care services: primary care provided by family doctors, emergency medical care, specialized (secondary and tertiary) medical care and nursing care. Services can only be provided by individuals or institutions operating as private legal entities: a limited liability company, a foundation or a private entrepreneur (Koppel et al., 2008). As shown in this case study, there is, therefore, an explicit intention to ensure that health care providers in Estonia are "autonomous".

The current study focuses on specialized care and on governance practices and challenges. Section 7.2 includes information on the hospital sector, the targets for hospitals and the master plan guiding the development of the network, as well as the legal basis for governance. Section 7.3 analyses the legal status of hospitals, the composition and role of Supervisory Boards, reporting and performance monitoring, and internal management structures and practices. The final section includes the discussion and main conclusions.

The present study builds on earlier reports, a large-scale survey conducted among hospital Supervisory and Management Board members in 2006 (Habicht, Aaviksoo & Koppel, 2006; Reinap et al. 2006; Habicht et al. 2006), informal meetings with hospital governors in past years and recent interviews conducted in 2009.[13]

7.2 Hospital sector in Estonia

Hospital sector reform in Estonia has been an important and integral part of overall health system restructuring. Looking at the set of objectives and measurable targets until now, the hospital sector reform has been relatively successful. The main driver of the accomplishment of set targets in the Hospital Master Plan (HMP) has been the structural changes in the hospital network due to the enforcement of the new Health Care Services Organization Act (Koppel et al., 2008; Palu & Kadakmaa, 2001). According to this legislation, all public hospitals had to be incorporated into private law as foundations or joint-stock companies, with full managerial rights over assets and access to financial markets, but at the same time giving them full residual claimant

---

13 To gain insight into the governance and management of Estonian hospitals, a semi-structured interview questionnaire was prepared in 2009, covering as the main areas of interest the legal status and role of the hospital; the mission, targets and reporting; along with financial management, internal structures and management of personnel. The questionnaire is available from the authors. The interviews were conducted with the managers of four specific hospitals (three included in the HMP and one private hospital in the capital region), as various types of information were already available from previous studies. The interviews were conducted by two people and recorded in the North Estonia Medical Centre (15 October 2009), Tartu University Clinic (10 November 2009), Pärnu Hospital (13 November 2009) and Fertilitas Private Clinic (21 October 2009). The current chapter uses reference interviews from 2009, although analyses also built on the key findings from earlier surveys.

status. In practice, this resulted in several hospital mergers and restructuring of services to achieve efficiency gains (Habicht & Habicht, 2008). Another important driver has been the EHIF's purchasing strategy, which has been targeting HMP objectives.

The regulatory environment for hospitals has been developed in line with health sector reforms. In 1991, the Health Insurance Act came into force as the basis for restructuring the Soviet-style health care system by introducing mandatory SHI. This act was followed by the Health Care Organization Act in 1994. With this legislation, the health service planning function was largely delegated to the municipality level, with the intention of decreasing the central government role. A providers' licensing system was also introduced – an important precondition for decreasing hospital network capacity and ensuring quality. In Estonia, the first system of hospital licensing was developed in 1994. According to that system, standards were developed for 26 types of specialist departments for laboratories, diagnostic and intensive care services. In addition, separate requirements were put in place for different levels of hospitals. A first round of hospital licensing was carried out at the end of 1994 (Jesse & Marshall, 1996). However, the legislation introduced was not particularly comprehensive and did not support the development of supervision and accountability. Moreover, where very different practices existed within the country, the municipalities were not as active as planned in taking forward their role as owners and governors.

Hospital governance in Estonia and how it has changed since the mid-1990s should be seen in an historical perspective. In the early 1990s, all hospitals were under state ownership, but the situation changed when both the Health Insurance Act and the Health Care Organization Act came into force in 1992 and 1994, respectively. According to the new framework, the Ministry of Social Affairs began to decentralize the hospital network. Most specialized tertiary hospitals (seven) remained directly under the Ministry of Social Affairs, while some were transferred to municipalities. Most other hospitals (general county and smaller long-term hospitals) were transferred to municipalities, with some exceptions in areas in which municipalities played a passive role. As a result, the decentralization was only implemented. The hospitals began operating using a variety of legal statuses.

In terms of management, prior to the implementation in 2002 of the new Health Services Organization Act, which clearly defined the legal status of hospitals and other health care institutions, there had been uncertainty regarding the autonomy of hospital managers. In the absence of legal requirements, some municipalities established hospitals as non-profit-making nongovernmental organizations, some as joint-stock companies and some as municipal agencies. In the 1990s, the Ministry of Social Affairs retained direct control of some tertiary and a few secondary hospitals that the municipalities had refused to take ownership of in 1994. These hospitals were legally defined as lower-level state agencies. Consequently, there was variation among hospitals in terms of managerial scope and accountability mechanisms. Although hospitals with state or municipal agency status had less managerial freedom than the other hospitals, in practice neither the Ministry of Social Affairs nor the municipalities were directly involved in managing them, and levels of accountability were low. There was no difference, however, in staff policies in the different hospitals from the beginning of 1990s. Medical professionals began working according to private labour regulations and were no longer part of the civil service in 1992 in all health institutions. Hospitals had the autonomy to develop salary policies and negotiate with individual staff members. The new Act clearly defined all providers as private entities operating under private law, with public interests represented through public membership of supervisory boards (Jesse et al., 2004).

As already discussed, by the late 1990s it was evident that the decentralization process was not efficient and the state started to recentralize more functions of hospital network planning (including the HMP) and governance. Decentralizing provider-related planning functions to the municipalities failed, as municipalities tend to protect the interests of local providers rather than targeting efficiency and accountability at system level. Also, the municipalities were very fragmented administrative units lacking the revenue base and competences to govern the health care sector. It thus became clear that some functions should be recentralized and the legal status of providers had to be clearly established, with the Ministry of Social Affairs taking a more active role in planning the network of providers.

The first step was preparation of the HMP 2015, to make projections regarding required future hospital capacity. A consultancy for the HMP was commissioned by the Ministry of Social Affairs, carried out by Swedish consultants and the results published in April 2000 (Jesse et al., 2004). Criteria used for planning hospital capacity included sufficient population pools (catchments areas) to support minimum service volumes for quality and efficiency, development of medical technology, demographic and epidemiological projections and a requirement that a hospital should not be further away than 60 minutes' travel time by car (70 km) (Ministry of Social Affairs, 1999). The plan suggested reducing the number of acute inpatient beds by two thirds and concentrating acute inpatient care in 15 larger hospitals, decreasing the total number of hospitals – through mergers and other types of restructuring – by three quarters (from 68 to 15) by 2015 (Ministry of Social Affairs, 1999).

Despite the negative publicity surrounding the HMP 2015, the Ministry of Social Affairs has used it as a basis for further discussion and it was an important trigger for further changes in the hospital sector. Principles listed in the HMP 2015 were taken as a basis and further outlined in the Health Services Organization Act, which was adopted in 2001. Thus, the structural and governance changes were simultaneously applied.

In addition, development plans by each county (15 regions in total) and by medical specialties were drawn up in 2001, which was the first time county doctors and specialist associations had formulated explicitly their long-term plans for health care. Based on these documents and the HMP 2015, the Ministry of Social Affairs elaborated and modified the HMP in 2002 (Ministry of Social Affairs, 2002; Bakler, 2003). After a series of consultations and some compromises, the extract of the HMP of 2002 was approved as government regulation in April 2003. The final version envisaged 19 hospitals (rather than 15, as suggested by consultants in a version of the HMP in 1999) as being eligible for long-term contracts with the EHIF and for state investment.

The new Health Services Organization Act was launched in 2001. The key changes set out in this Act included recentralizing planning functions at the national level, establishing a new licensing system for both doctors and providers, defining the legal status of providers as private entities, and explicitly defining the financing responsibilities of different sources of funding. In 2002, the new Health Services Organization Act came into force, establishing the Health Care Board as a separate state agency for licensing providers and supervising the health system (Jesse et al., 2004; Koppel et al., 2008).

The Act defined seven types of hospital in Estonia: regional hospital, central hospital, general hospital, local hospital, special hospital, rehabilitation hospital and nursing hospital, of which the first four are acute-care hospitals. For each type of hospital there are special requirements established by the Ministry of Social Affairs, such as the list and scale of services to be provided and standards for the rooms, medical equipment and medical staff. In 2005, each hospital was required to obtain an activity licence according to the hospital type, lasting for five years. The licensing system and minimum standards for hospitals are now fully operational in Estonia. According to the results of a postal survey and interviews conducted in 2006 with key informants, hospital managers found that even current regulations (requirements for hospital types) are too restrictive and inflexible, which results in inefficient use of resources. This refers to the perception of the managers in settings in which even higher autonomy is expected, which launches a debate on autonomy and accountability.

In spring 2003, the government approved the Hospital Network Development Plan based on the principles of the above-mentioned HMP 2002. In order to ensure equality in terms of availability of specialist medical services, the plan foresees 19 active treatment hospitals. The list of hospitals includes 12 general and local hospitals, 4 central hospitals and 3 regional hospitals (see Fig. 7.1).

Fig. 7.1 *Acute-care hospital network in Estonia, 2009*

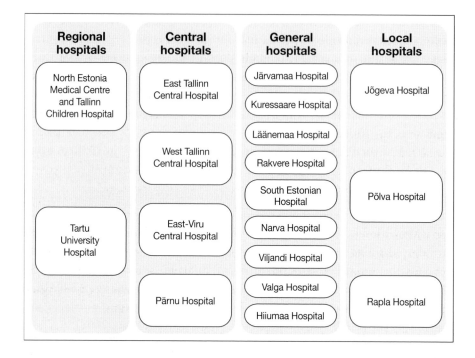

Three regional hospitals in Estonia provide about 33% of total bed capacity. Two regional hospitals (secondary and tertiary care), the North Estonian Regional Hospital and the Tartu University Hospital, are the largest hospitals and each serves an area with about 500 000 population. The third regional hospital, Tallinn Children Hospital, provides medical services at the highest level to children living in north and west Estonia. There are four central hospitals (23% of the total number of beds), each serving a catchment area of about 200 000 people and providing mainly secondary care, along with some tertiary care.

Local and general hospitals (with 5% and 24% of total bed capacity, respectively) are small active treatment hospitals, most with 50–200 beds, providing treatment for common diseases closest to where people live. There is at least one local or general hospital in each Estonian county. The local hospitals are necessary in centres situated at a distance of more than 70 km from a general, central or regional hospital, or in county centres (Koppel et al., 2008). The exceptions for general hospitals are Tartu, Pärnu and Harju County where, according to the Hospital Network Development Plan, there will be no separate general hospital, with these services instead being provided by a central or regional hospital.

The new Health Care Services Organization Act was intended to harmonize the legal basis for hospitals; all public hospitals providing inpatient and/or outpatient care were required to be incorporated into private law as foundations or joint-stock companies. This means that all public hospitals must operate under the Foundations Act (as foundations) or under the Commercial Code (as joint-stock companies). Both acts set the general rules for these legal forms, without any special regulation for the hospital sector (thus applicable for all sectors in Estonia). Although there are no large legal differences between joint-stock companies (regulated by the Commercial Code) and foundations (regulated by the Foundations Act) in terms of running a hospital, both types nonetheless have some limited specific features. In 2008, about 60% of hospitals – including 70% of all bed capacity – were already "foundations".

It was foreseen that each type of organization should have a Supervisory Board and a Management Board. The responsibility of the former would be strategic planning and supervision over the latter, which was responsible for running the hospital according to Supervisory Board guidance. Each hospital would be allowed to specify in detail further organizational issues, including governance practices and responsibilities in the individual hospital's statutes.

The total number of hospitals in Estonia is 60, of which 38 are owned by the state or local municipalities, representing 90% of the total number of hospital beds. The number of acute-care hospitals has decreased dramatically since the early 1990s, from 118 in 1992 to 37 in 2008. There have been two major reductions in the number of acute-care hospitals, as described earlier. First, in the mid-1990s, hospital licensing was introduced and, as a result, some small providers were not able to fulfil the criteria. Some of these providers supply predominantly long-term care (as nursing homes, for example), or were transformed into outpatient centres. Second, a fall in numbers took place at the beginning of this century, related to the hospital mergers. In recent years, the number of hospitals has been increasing slightly, specifically due to an increase in specialized care hospitals.

In 2009, the National Audit Office of Estonia conducted an assessment of the achievement of hospital sector restructuring targets, as well as current strengths and weaknesses, while simultaneously providing proposals for further infrastructure improvement (National Audit Office of Estonia, 2010). A call for further changes in the hospital sector – both in terms of infrastructure and clinical practices – is highlighted in a recent analysis of the sustainability of the health financing system in Estonia (Thomson et al., 2010).

7.3 Governance mechanisms in the Estonian hospital sector

7.3.1 Institutional arrangements

Legal form and objectives

The current organization of hospital governance is universally defined and transparent in Estonia (see Fig. 7.2). Both legal entities (that is, joint-stock companies and foundations) must have a Supervisory Board as the governing body and a Management Board for day-to-day operations. The responsibilities of these bodies are outlined in more detail in the case of limited-stock companies. In addition, more detailed tasks and responsibilities can be set out in the organizations' statutes.

Fig. 7.2 *Hospitals' governance structure in Estonia*

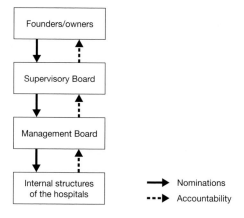

Hospital ownership is one important aspect of legal status. In the case of joint-stock companies, shareholders own the hospital. In the case of foundations, there is no mention of an "owner" but rather a "founder", perhaps mainly a semantic difference indicating a weaker "sense of ownership" in the case of foundations. The weak role and liability of owners (or founders) was one of the most frequently mentioned problems during the aforementioned interviews with managers conducted in 2006.

In Estonia, most hospitals are owned (or founded) by the state, the local governments or some public legal bodies (for example, the University of Tartu). There are usually multiple owners (for example, the central state and the local municipalities jointly owning one hospital, or a number of local municipalities owning one hospital). Multiple ownership weakens the owners' motivation to take responsibility, also expressed as less willingness to invest in the hospital. The fact that most hospital revenue is generated through the contract with the EHIF is also relevant; as contracts are negotiated with the hospital's Management Board, the owners' role is only marginal.

Another issue related to the legal status of hospitals in the respective cases of a foundation and a joint-stock company is the organization's objective. A joint-stock company is understood to be a business organization, and so maximizing profits should be its main objective. However, some actors do not perceive this to be an acceptable objective for publicly owned hospitals, and some opinion leaders do not consider a joint-stock company to be a suitable legal status for hospitals (Reinap et al., 2006). Accordingly, one difference between a foundation and a joint-stock company is that financial supervision is much stricter in the case of joint-stock companies.

Although there is no legal provision that a joint-stock company should maximize profit but rather "act in an economically reasonably way", somehow the joint-stock company status is automatically translated into a profit-making obligation. One of the concerns about joint-stock companies is that they will become profit maximizers, to the extent that other objectives (such as social issues) would become less important. However, in the hospital managers survey in 2006 it was clearly pointed out that joint-stock companies in the health sector would have other objectives than maximizing profit if such was the will of their owners. That is, if owners were to represent perfectly public interests, the legal status of hospitals would not be a restricting factor. A particular threat perceived in the current system is that hospitals could decide to reinvest their profits outside the health care sector; however, this is a theoretical risk, rather than an actual threat.

In summary, there seems to be lack of common understanding of hospitals' objectives. How do we recognize a hospital that is performing well? How do different legal forms actually function and how do they enable hospitals to achieve their objectives? Even if the regulatory hospital governance structure is set up and enforced, a common understanding of what this really means is still evolving and would need further institutionalization. This may be the result of poor information sharing and guidance on how to govern the hospital sector – an argument supported by the results of the postal survey in 2006 (Habicht et al., 2006), according to which most Supervisory Board members (61%) replied that the Ministry of Social Affairs "should give them more guidance on how to govern hospitals", such as best practice guidelines and training for both Management Board and Supervisory Board members.

Follow-up interviews in 2009 highlighted that there has been no real consideration of a change of legal status, although there have been debates regarding legal forms. The possibility of a specific legal status for the hospital sector was considered in the mid-1990s and once again in 2005, but the current overall private sector legislation was found to be suitable after discussing pros and cons. Currently, the main limitation mentioned by managers in foundations is restricted access to local development funds and research grants. Merging institutions would also become easier if all hospitals had the same legal status, but this specifically has not been an obstacle for changes thus far. Hospital managers see foundations as a more stable organizational form than joint-stock companies. It was also pointed out that foundations seem to have a more positive and accepted image among the general public and health care workers than the organizations with joint-stock company status.

Room for decisions

Decisions relating to the internal structure of the hospitals are mostly the domain of Management Boards. The need to redefine hospital legal status in 2002 gave hospitals an opportunity to reconsider the extent of decentralization of the current management structures, the delegation of decision rights to structural units and the scope of structural units' budgets. As could be expected, more changes occurred in hospitals that were merged into bigger hospitals, with fewer changes occurring in those hospitals that only changed their legal status.

Relations with stakeholders, role of professional organizations and unions

The role of stakeholders and professional organizations is stronger in developing and consulting on health policy initiatives at national level, including policies on principles of regulation, planning and financing hospital services. At hospital management level, the role of professional organizations is limited. The unions of health care professionals play an important role, together with the Hospital Union, in negotiating national-level agreements that set minimum remuneration levels for health professionals, as well as at the level of the individual hospitals, in negotiations of collective agreements at hospital level.

The EHIF does not participate in hospital governing bodies. Hospitals' relations with the EHIF are only based on contractual agreements.

7.3.2 Financial arrangements

Estonian hospitals have residual claimant status, that is, they can keep the revenue earned and are responsible for covering possible short-falls, and there is no difference between the different legal types.

Hospitals' annual budgets are prepared by their Management Boards and are approved by their Supervisory Boards. Their revenue consists mostly of funds from the EHIF for reimbursement of services provided to insured individuals and emergency care for the uninsured population. Hospitals have the right to establish co-payments for specialist ambulatory visits and individual bed days, up to a maximum per visit and per bed day, as regulated by law. These form a marginal proportion of the total revenue and are not earmarked for specific expenditures. Some hospitals allow their "structural units" to retain earnings for services paid privately, and doctors and nurses can also be paid bonuses from these earnings. In addition, some hospitals provide laboratory and diagnostic services for other health care providers, such as primary care centres. All hospitals are entitled to retain any surplus and to reinvest it into the infrastructure or equipment. Hospitals acting as joint-stock companies have the right to pay dividends to shareholders, but this right has not been used yet by any, as in case of public hospitals the shareholders are municipalities, not private investors.

Where central drug registers have been put in place, pharmaceutical studies represent another source of additional revenue (some of the revenue is pooled at hospital level and other funds are retained by the investigating doctor). The financial crisis has increased awareness among managers about how and where additional revenue for the hospital could be obtained.

Hospitals operating as foundations are subject to public procurement law and have recruited procurement specialists who are responsible for conducting the procurement process. Specifications and evaluations are carried out by specific committees, members of which are required to state in writing that there is no conflict of interest related to the procurement undertaking in question.

Hospitals are responsible for the planning of investments. Most hospitals develop specific long-term investment plans and set up financial mechanisms to fund these. Hospitals are permitted to borrow, as well as to use other financial instruments to finance investments. The more decentralized hospitals (see subsection 7.3.4) started out with some of the revenue for investments and decisions remaining at the clinic level. Over time, the hospital discussed in the example centralized investment planning, with the Management Board prioritizing investment proposals in the investment plan, which is approved by the Supervisory Board. The other hospitals have become more decentralized in their evolution: the Supervisory Board decides upon allocation for investment and the clinics prepare their investment programmes within the ceilings set by the Management Board. In both regional hospitals, investment priorities have depended upon the need for renovations using EU Regional Development Fund financing since 2007.

In smaller hospitals, structural units or departments are responsible for the budgets for salaries and consumables, with most decisions being made at Management Board level. In larger hospitals, some of the revenue for small-scale investments and decisions remain at the level of structural units, while larger-scale investments are decided by Management Boards and also by Supervisory Boards.

7.3.3 Accountability arrangements

Supervisory Board

The main responsibilities of the Supervisory Board are described in their respective legal acts and hospital statutes. As already mentioned, most hospitals in Estonia are owned by the state or local governments. Therefore, nominated Supervisory Board members have a political mandate (and quite frequently a political background as well). This led to discussion of the extent of politicization of hospitals' governance structures and its influence on hospital performance. While previously directly managed by the Ministry of Social Affairs or municipal agencies, the hospital sector was not a priority – it was considered merely a medical domain and politicians rarely took interest in it for that reason. According to the results of a Supervisory Board members' postal survey in 2006 (Habicht et al., 2006), some 69% of respondents considered Supervisory Boards to be over-politicized. Exactly the same proportion of respondents agreed that in order to guarantee the fulfilment of owners' or founders' interests, Supervisory Boards should be professional rather than political.

In the current governance structure, it seems inevitable that Supervisory Boards are to some extent politicized and this is not seen by different stakeholders as being a major problem, other than if and when this starts to influence management and other staff beyond reason, and if managers are selected not by taking into account competence and experience, but rather by considering political suitability. Both issues were highlighted in the 2006 survey and the interviews in 2009.

There seems to be common understanding of the Supervisory Board's role(s) according to the survey results: strategy building, supervision of managers and financial issues. Yet, some 69% of Supervisory Board members expressed the belief in 2006 (Habicht et al., 2006) that the Supervisory Board should have a more significant role. It is worth noting that the situation has improved over the years, even though at the beginning the Supervisory Board's role was minimal. This is due to an accumulation of experience, since the creation of Supervisory Boards, in steering hospitals via board structures.

According to the results of the same survey, there is room for improvement in the performance of the Supervisory Boards, although first there is a need to agree on what are good performance criteria (for example, one answer during the 2006 interviews was: "Supervisory Boards' performance is good and they haven't disturbed hospitals' development" (Habicht et al., 2006)).

The selection process for Supervisory Board members may be related to poor board performance. Usually, government agencies or city council members are nominated and most members have a political mandate, which means there is no guarantee that nominated members will have the necessary competences to provide strategic stewardship required for the hospital sector. A political mandate also means that if there are changes in political power, changes in Supervisory Board composition will tend to follow suit. Therefore, Supervisory Boards in Estonia have had relatively high turnover. In the 2006 postal survey (Habicht et al., 2006), most of the members of HMP hospitals' Supervisory Boards (92%) agreed with the statement that "Supervisory Board members change too frequently in Estonia and this affects adversely the sustainability of the boards' activity".

Mixed representation in the Supervisory Boards could increase continuity, thus offering a means of avoiding the connection between Supervisory Board membership and political electoral cycles. An example is the Tartu University Hospital Supervisory Board, of which both Tartu City and State (in addition to the University of Tartu as a third party) are the founders. Due to different electoral cycles at national and local levels, changes of nominated members in the Supervisory Board usually do not take place in the same year, ensuring greater stability. The hospital managers highlighted in 2009 that stability guaranteed by such composition is beneficial for sustainable hospital development. In addition, bringing in different stakeholders to the hospital governance structure ensures a balance of interests over time. Having the informal agreement of the owner to appoint a number of non-political Supervisory Board members (three out of seven) representing health sector competences at national and local levels is another potential alternative, as demonstrated in Pärnu Hospital. It is also clear that practices in the private clinics are different, where the Supervisory Board members are hospital investors and a much closer relationship exists in clinic governance structures.

In the current system, there is limited support for Supervisory Board members in terms of guidance and advice. There is also limited use of outside hospital expertise to support decision-making processes. In order to increase the role of the Supervisory Boards in governing hospitals, the EHIF holds regular meetings since 2008 with the Supervisory Boards in each hospital, sharing current performance information and the offering the opinion(s) of the purchaser.

This has increased understanding of the strategic role of Supervisory Boards in some hospitals.

Some options to further improve Supervisory Boards' performance in Estonia are explored here. One possibility is to set strict requirements (for example, educational background) for Supervisory Board members within legal acts. The downside to this approach is that it is very difficult to set objective criteria that actually guarantee the competence of board members, and this option has not found any support. This option was debated among decision-makers a few years ago in Estonia and found not to be suitable at the time. A second option is to prepare a code of conduct for Supervisory Board members, which helps to determine the hospital's culture. A third option that has been mentioned is to offer training and coaching (which might be mandatory) to enable Supervisory Board members to improve their competences.

Public reporting, oversight and performance monitoring

Public accountability within the hospital can be exercised if objectives have been set for the hospital to which hospital managers can be held accountable. Such objectives are usually set in accordance with longer-term strategic development, including the wording of the vision and mission statement. All Estonian central and regional hospitals now have a clear vision and mission statements, as well as development and business plans, although the content of the latter varies (Habicht, Aaviksoo & Koppel, 2006). One question relates to the differences in the matters emphasized by Supervisory Board members and managers. The results from 2006 show differences in the priority afforded to investment in quality of services and access to care – while Supervisory Board members see access to care as the most important issue, hospital managers ranked this as only fifth, prioritizing instead investment in the quality of care. There were no significant differences concerning other objectives, such as improving client services, increasing efficiency, developing new services and increasing market share (Habicht, Aaviksoo & Koppel, 2006). The same study highlighted that the actual decisions made do not always follow the strategic directions that have been outlined, and this could be improved. This can be explained by a finding in the interviews conducted in 2009 – practice varies between hospitals in terms of using their development plans as planning and accountability tools. In some hospitals, the development plan is a tool which is reviewed, monitored and updated annually. In others, the development plan is more general and is not subject to annual review to measure progress.

A study analysing the culture of performance measurement and management in large hospitals in 2009 (Guisset, Kjaergaard & Habicht, 2009) highlighted that recently the emphasis of the hospitals' governance has been focused on efficiency measures and restructuring. During recent years, scrutiny on the part of Supervisory Boards and Management Boards has focused more on the volume and prices of services (content of the contracts with the EHIF) and patient satisfaction (patient complaints, essentially), reflecting the measurement focus in the context of hospital reforms. There are observable discrepancies between strategic statements, performance measurement and internal accountability structures in hospitals, highlighting the need for development on two levels. On one level, there are opportunities to create additional external pressures in order to bring stakeholders more closely together and create strong incentives for comprehensive performance management. On the other level, there is potential to build on the numerous initiatives already being implemented and the good practices available within individual hospitals.

The extent of external accountability can be measured by what performance and management information is publicized by the hospitals, as well as by statements regarding to whom hospital managers feel primarily accountable. A varying degree of transparency could be observed in a review of the Internet home pages of the four hospitals interviewed for the current study in September 2009 – not all had published their development plans, annual action plans, annual reports, or even budgets with explanatory notes.

While there are clearly defined systems for planning, reporting and performance measurement, the question arises regarding to whom managers personally feel most accountable. Some managers feel that the top priority (for accountability) is their workers ("most of my working time is allocated to employees in my hospital; if health care workers are satisfied they also provide higher quality services"), followed by the EHIF as purchaser and the Supervisory Board. Other managers feel that the highest priority is doctors and nurses, followed by patients and the Supervisory Board. A third hospital mentioned the Supervisory Board, representing the owners, followed by the purchaser (who also represents patients through their contracts) and employees.

The role and activity of the Supervisory Board vary, but they seem to have a clear role in terms of discussing and approving the long-term, mid-range and annual action plans, including clear targets. Hospitals also differ in their use of quantitative and qualitative targets in action plans to be measured at the end of the period. As the overall health system is changing, how the mission statements are changing over time was also mentioned in one interview. Some years ago, the emphasis was on being the best, essentially declaring competition between the hospitals. As the roles of hospitals have become clearer, mission statements have also started to emphasize more the role within the care network and cooperation between hospitals.

Meetings (varying from quarterly to monthly) and reporting to the Supervisory Board are regular activities in all the hospitals interviewed. Over the years, the topics and depth of discussions have varied, depending on personalities of the board members, their previous experience with the health sector and their interests. Reporting has received more attention over the years, with priority being afforded to financial reporting, derived as a responsibility from their autonomy and legal status. As hospitals are legal entities, their annual reports are audited by independent auditors. This has influenced the content of hospitals' annual reports, which have become more oriented towards financial performance and the achievement of the HMP targets.

7.3.4 Internal management structures and functions

Decisions relating to the internal structure of the hospitals are mostly the domain of Management Boards. The need to redefine hospital legal status in 2002 provided an opportunity for managers to reconsider the extent of decentralization of the current management structures, the delegation of decision rights to structural units and the scope of structural units' budgets. In the hospitals which only changed their legal status, fewer changes occurred, while more changes took place in hospitals which were merged into larger hospitals.

Approaches taken in hospital merger cases have varied, with the two regional hospitals described here providing examples from opposite ends of the centralization/decentralization spectrum.

One of these regional hospitals, established in 1999, opted for a decentralized structure; the 1300-bed hospital operated across 19 separate buildings (some of which were several kilometres apart) and implemented an internal structure based on 17 clinics, with most decision rights delegated to the heads of clinics. The clinics were viewed as revenue-generating units, with budgets dependent on revenue earned. The change brought about different influences from the previous structure, as for most clinics the planning and monitoring of financial performance at clinic level was a new approach, while some saw their rights restricted. Establishing internal reimbursement for services provided to other clinics was also under consideration. The Management Board's role is now to monitor individual clinics' performance and to ensure resource allocations between them, as some specialties have greater opportunity to generate revenue.

The other regional hospital – a 1500-bed hospital operating across 15 facilities at the time of the merger – opted for a much narrower structure, with only four clinics in charge of budget and administrative issues. Considerably more decisions were retained at the Management Board level during the initial years, with plans to devolve these more after the merger process had been completed.

Over 10 years later, the structures and processes of the two hospitals have not converged significantly; one remains more decentralized and the other one remains fairly centralized. The respective hospital managers highlighted in the interviews the strengths of their chosen options – ease of responding to pressures in times of financial crises in the case of more centralized structures and shared accountability in more de-centralized settings. This demonstrates that both management (centralization) variants can be made to work. Some functions have been centralized in both regional hospitals – namely, procurement of high-cost equipment and high-volume consumables.

As an example, a 390-bed central hospital used the decentralized model initially, but over the years has centralized some functions back to the Management Board level. The main reason for this was said to be lack of good-quality mid-level managers who were able to perform well in terms of their administrative duties as well as clinical practice in a smaller hospital setting.

The development of clinical specialties is defined by the type of hospital and the licensing process, which does not restrict hospitals from developing some areas more than others. So far there are no specific strategies developed for clinical areas in the hospitals interviewed under public ownership. However, in all hospitals there are cases in which some specialties have been faster in their development – something mostly attributed in the interviews with hospital managers to the existence of a visionary clinical leader in the field, as well to the availability of new medical technology. The practice contrasted with that of the private clinic, for which very clear criteria were set by hospital management when selecting, opening or scaling up any clinical specialty. The difference included clearly set priorities regarding what should be the core specialties and which clinical or practice areas could be supported.

Regarding remuneration policies, hospitals have specific remuneration policies, with basic salary scales allocated according to staff category. The remuneration policies in the Estonian hospital sector are available to hospital staff but individual salaries are confidential, with the exception of those of the members of Management Boards, which are made available on hospital web sites.

Minimum wage agreements to be followed at hospital level are concluded at state level. The different coefficients for basic salaries are applied at provider level, depending on speciality and on hospital priorities. This results in almost twice the income differences in medical doctors at the same level from different specialties within one hospital. Salaries for nurses across different units within the hospital are more equal. In the past it has been customary also to use performance-related pay as part of the salary structure. The share of performance-related pay reached over 50% in private clinics; less in public hospitals. Performance-related pay is mostly applied to doctors and less often to nurses – its impact on the salary structure also differs between specialties and clinics within one hospital. In response to decreasing revenues resulting from the financial crisis, hospitals decreased or omitted individuals' performance-based pay during 2009. While the salary policy is accessible to staff, individual salaries are confidential.

7.4 Discussion and conclusions

Since the early 1990s, the Estonian hospital sector has changed from a centrally planned, directly managed and norm-based financed model into a sector in which revenue and doctors' income depend on workload and related considerations.

The extent of changes has also caused governance mechanisms to undergo fundamental changes in order to ensure that hospitals fulfil public expectations and interests; current governance structures have evolved over time, drawing on experience from within the health sector, among others. An important factor in this regard has been timeliness in addressing deficiencies or problems experienced. Hospitals have a substantial degree of autonomy to decide upon their structure, expenditure, recruitment and investment, among other things.

The current experience can be summarized in the following points.

- The governance structures for hospitals were harmonized in 2002, introducing two-tier governance structures (Supervisory Board and Management Board) and two legal forms (foundation and joint-stock company). While this has clarified the framework, practices vary between and within hospitals to a certain extent.

- The roles and responsibilities for both Supervisory and Management Boards are defined in hospital statutes, although variation between providers is rather minimal and standard approaches are applied.

- Public sector oversight of hospital activities (as owner) depends on how Supervisory Boards perform. Performance is influenced by the Boards' composition (which determines their competence and stability over time), as well as by representation of the health system and central or local political vision. From qualitative surveys and interviews we may conclude that Supervisory Boards with broader representation balancing political and non-political representation perform better and are more stable over time.

- Differences in governance, performance and management cannot be explained by legal status (whether foundation or joint-stock company). The different forms encompass variations in how the new hospital is formed, but this plays a marginal role for HMP hospitals, as they are former public hospitals. While some legal differences exist, their impact is for the most part intangible, as foundations have a better image among health care professionals and the public.

- The differences in performance are linked to how well the Management Board performs and how well the Supervisory Board guides and oversees the hospital's strategic issues. This also includes the selection of board members and the reaction of supervisors to the Management Boards that are not performing well over the years.

- Supervisory Boards have tended to focus more on financial aspects, with increasing interest in quality of care and especially access to care. Over time, Management Boards have initiated several performance measurement exercises.

- The most strategic decisions of the Supervisory Boards comprise the selection of Management Boards, setting their objectives and overseeing their fulfilment. The Estonian experience has been that, when extensive structural changes have been required, Supervisory Boards have selected Management Board members from outside the hospital, both from within the health sector and externally. Those managers have introduced new management practices within hospitals and have been able to manage organizational change more effectively. Reasons for changing Management Board members have included poor performance and in some cases political influences.

- The current governance and management practices within hospitals vary, but that variation is for the most part not as a result of the legal form or Supervisory Board composition, but rather of the composition and competences of the Management Board, internal structures of the hospital and the balance of power between managers and health care professionals.

- Internal structures and decision rights of structural units depend on both the size of the hospital and past decisions relating to structure. As expected, smaller hospitals have more centralized managerial decision-making in terms of budgets, procurement, and so on.

- All hospitals have centralized investment decisions and the procurement of high-cost equipment or high-volume consumables.

- Interviews revealed that defining priorities for clinical development and for the adoption of new services is mostly dependent on visionary clinical leaders, rather than the Supervisory Board. The EHIF meets annually with each hospital Supervisory Board in order to provide them with external feedback on performance and additional input in terms of setting objectives.

In conclusion, the Estonian experience shows that the hospital sector governance set-up should be aligned with governance of other sectors, as the legal framework is also applied to primary care practices. Moreover, the same models have been used in the social sector, education and other public services, such as the postal service, national energy companies and municipal transport services. This makes it possible to draw on lessons learned and expertise from other parts of the social and industrial economy. Governance is a process in which constant learning is essential and the importance of addressing timely emerging problems is clear.

7.5 References

Bakler T (2003). "Hospital master Plan´ist" haiglavõrgu arengukavani. [From "hospital masterplan" to hospital development plan]. *Eesti Arst*, (Special issue):23–27.

Guisset A-L, Kjaergaard J, Habicht J (2009). *Performance management, developing a culture of measurement and continuous quality improvement in Estonian hospitals: recommendations on alternative entry points and ways forward.* Copenhagen, WHO Regional Office for Europe.

Habicht T (2008). Governing a single-payer mandatory health insurance system: the case of Estonia. In: Sawedoff WD, Gottret P, eds. *Governing mandatory health insurance. Learning from experience.* Washington, DC, World Bank:101–128.

Habicht T, Habicht J (2008). Estonia: "good practice" in expanding health care coverage. In: Gottret P, Schieber GJ, Waters H, eds. *Good practices in health financing: lessons from reforms in low and middle-income countries.* Washington, DC, World Bank:227–267.

Habicht T, Aaviksoo A, Koppel A (2006). *Hospital sector reform in Estonia: summary.* Tallinn, PRAXIS Center for Policy Studies.

Habicht T et al. (2006). *The study on the impact of the Estonian health reform. Report based on the questionnaire for hospital supervisory board members.* Tallinn, PRAXIS Center for Policy Studies.

Jesse M, Marshall T (1996). *Health care systems in transition: Estonia.* Copenhagen, WHO Regional Office for Europe.

Jesse M et al. (2004). *Health care systems in transition: Estonia.* Copenhagen, WHO Regional Office for Europe on behalf of the European Observatory on Health Systems and Policies.

Koppel A et al. (2008). Estonia: health system review. *Health Systems in Transition*, 10(1):1–230.

Ministry of Social Affairs (1999). *Estonian hospital master plan 2015*. Tallinn, Ministry of Social Affairs.

Ministry of Social Affairs (2002) *Eesti Haiglavõrgu Arengukava [The hospital network development plan]*. Tallinn, Ministry of Social Affairs.

National Audit Office of Estonia (2010). *Haiglavõrgu jätkusuutlikkus [The sustainability of hospital network]*. Tallinn, National Audit Office of Estonia. (Report of the National Audit Office to the Riigikogu).

Palu T, Kadakmaa R (2001). Estonian hospital sector in transition. *Eurohealth*, 7(3)(Special Issue).

Reinap M et al. (2006). *The study on the impact of the Estonian health reform. Report based on the questionnaire for hospital management board members. Summary*. Tallinn, Praxis Center for Policy Studies.

Thomson S et al. (2010). *Responding to the challenge of financial sustainability in Estonia's health system*. Copenhagen, WHO Regional Office for Europe.

Chapter 8
Israel

David Chinitz[14]

8.1 Introduction

Israel's health system is pluralistic, meaning that services are financed and provided by multiple sectors, including government, voluntary non-profit-making and private agents. This pluralistic structure has, over time, become subject to greater government regulation. Since 1995, four non-profit-making sickness funds, or health plans, which previously provided uneven, segmented coverage, are now required – under the National Health Insurance Law – to provide a standard "basket" of services. The health plans do not charge premiums directly to citizens, who instead pay an earmarked health tax to the National Insurance Institute. Government supplements the financing of the standard basket of services with budgets derived from general tax revenues. In addition, the system is financed by co-payments and various forms of supplemental insurance. Overall, health expenditure accounts for about 8% of gross domestic product (Bennun, Berlowitz & Shani, 2005; Rosen, 2009).

The health plans receive an age-adjusted, capitated budget, paid to them by the government. Citizens are free to switch between the funds several times annually, without restriction. The sickness funds are able to selectively contract with providers, including primary care physicians and specialists working in the community and hospitals, and in so doing compete for enrolees (Rosen, 2009). The health plans have strong networks of primary care physicians; however,

This chapter was based, in part, on interviews with and comments from hospital directors and other key informants. I thank Dr Eran Halpern, Professor Yair Shapira, Dr Rachelle Kaye and Professor Shlomo Mor Yosef for their contributions. Responsibility lies fully with the author.

citizens may also self-refer to community-based specialists and hospital outpatient departments.

General hospitals are owned by government (under the aegis of the Ministry of Health), sickness funds and non-profit-making associations. The Ministry of Health, together with the Ministry of Finance, suggests reimbursement rates to parliament, which – once approved – serve as benchmarks for the hospital system. This (among other factors) represents a conflict of interest for the government, as it can set conditions to the advantage of its own hospitals. Therefore, reform suggestions have been put forward, especially since 1995, aiming to convert government hospitals into independent trusts. This reform has not been implemented. However, the spectre of the reform has had an effect (Ministry of Health, 2002; [Anonymous] 2004; Feder-Bubis, 2006; Chinitz & Rosen, 1993).

8.2 Common governance features

Before exploring the specific cases, it is worthwhile mentioning some of the common governance features that apply to all the hospitals. First, all of the hospitals are subject to all relevant government legislation and public service regulations, in particular the Public Health Ordinance (State of Israel, 1940), first instituted during the British Mandate in 1940, which (among other things) provides the basis for licensing of medical institutions in the country. This statute governs the granting of hospital credentials and determines the medical fields that must be included in the hospitals' basket of services. All general hospitals are required to include certain basic services and departments: internal medicine, orthopaedics, obstetrics and gynaecology, and general surgery. Hospitals are required to obtain Ministry of Health approval for an increase in bed numbers, as well as the purchase and operation of certain equipment, such as MRI equipment. Minimum staffing levels are determined by the Ministry of Health, together with the various professional associations. A particular set of statutes, enacted in 2002 are the Health Corporation Regulations, which regulate hospital activities that operate outside the publicly budgeted financial structure of the hospital (State of Israel, 2002). The enactment and significance of these regulations are discussed in the case studies explored in the sections that follow. Finally, in addition to revenue from the sale of services to the health plans, all hospitals obtain some revenue from sources such as the National Insurance Institute (for birthing mothers), road accident insurance, services provided to military personnel, and medical tourism.

Consequently, when considering the hospitals reported on in this chapter, it is difficult to define ownership status, the degree to which there is separation between purchaser and provider, and between regulator and provider.

Israel has four main types of general hospital, as detailed here.

- Government-owned hospitals, with about 46% of the total beds, are owned, budgeted and operated by the Ministry of Health, with salaried employees paid by government.

- Sick fund-owned hospitals, with about 30% of the total beds, are owned, budgeted and operated by the sick funds, with salaried employees paid by the sick fund.

- Independent, non-profit-making hospitals, with about 19% of the total beds (all in Jerusalem), are owned by charitable organizations, financed based on the revenue they generate from selling services, and independently operated.

- Privately owned hospitals, with about 5% of the total beds are owned by shareholders and are independently operated.

However, this categorization is now inadequate, since one of the sick funds now owns and operates its own "private" hospitals, and another is a partner in a private hospital.

One result of this blurring of boundaries is that hospitals appear simultaneously to be on the one hand completely constrained by central government mandates and limitations and on the other have a high level of autonomy. This obviously complicates the governance picture. I return to these issues in section 8.7.

In this chapter, I discuss four hospitals, one that is government owned, one independent, one owned by a sick fund, and the new sick fund-owned private hospital. Two large general hospitals are described in terms of the questions posed in the briefing paper for this project. One of the hospitals is a large voluntary non-profit-making institution, while the other is of similar size, but owned by the government (specifically the Ministry of Health). Some educated first impressions are provided relating to the other two hospitals, demonstrating the rich variety represented by the cases. Israeli hospital governance is illustrative of blurred boundaries and a system with a combination of highly regulated parts, together with extremely autonomous ones. The advantages, disadvantages and viability of such a framework are explored in more detail throughout.[15]

---

15 The descriptions that follow are based on the author's own knowledge, research and discussions with experts, existing descriptions of the Israeli hospital system, and media reports.

8.3 Case study 1: a large non-profit-making hospital in Jerusalem

8.3.1 Strategic governance issues

Structural institutional framework

The hospital is required to provide certain basic departments, such as internal medicine, orthopaedics, paediatrics, obstetrics and gynaecology, and general surgery. However, due to its history, founded well before the state, along with its university affiliation, the hospital views itself (and others view it) as being expected to provide the highest level of tertiary care. So, in addition to departments such as cardiology, psychiatry, urology, oncology (including radiation) and bone marrow transplantation, the hospital provides sophisticated diagnostic services, such as MRI and positron emission tomography, transplantation surgery and neurosurgery. Moreover, the hospital is a major trauma treatment and emergency medicine hospital, which – given the Israeli security situation – establishes the hospital as one of the country leaders in these fields.

The decision to provide high-level tertiary services is in the hands of the Directorate of the hospital, subject to the approval of its owner (a United States-based Jewish Women's Organization (JWO)) and the approval of the Ministry of Health. If the Directorate decides to pursue a new initiative, such as purchase of an MRI scanner, either of these two agents – one an internal governance structure and the other an external regulatory body – may intervene, especially the latter. However, generally speaking, the hospital Directorate has considerable latitude in terms of such investments.

Within the hospital, department directors, who are very powerful actors, often propose new services, sometimes based around the acquisition of new technology; the Directorate evaluates the benefits and costs to the hospital and – if the project is found to be desirable – gives its approval. In addition, the hospital (with the implicit backing of the JWO) creates a centre based on existing services, such as the hospital's Mother and Child Center. This requires the approval of the Ministry of Health.

Financial framework

The conditions for the employment of physicians and nurses, and minimum staffing levels (number of staff per patient bed), are determined nationally in a set of negotiations and national collective agreements involving the Ministry of Health, the Ministry of Finance, the Israel Medical Association, and the unions representing physicians and nurses. These are salaried employees. The hospital, however, is permitted (due to historical precedent) to offer private medical services, which enable the patient to choose a physician for a consultation or procedure. The private service provides the opportunity for physicians and the hospital to garner additional revenue. By law, the hospital is not allowed to earn more than a certain percentage of its revenue from this source, and physicians receive only 19% of the payments made by patients in pre-payroll tax income.

Investment capital is provided by contributions, mostly from the JWO. While the JWO provides only about 10% of the budget, it also helps with raising contributions from major philanthropists. The hospital has also combined revenue raising with physical expansion, by renting out space for consumer-oriented activities, such as dedicating land to a shopping mall contiguous with the hospital. These kinds of expansions are initiated and approved by the Directorate, subject to approval by the Board. Funds for new equipment are usually also provided through contributions. Officially, the hospital needs Ministry of Health approval for this, but it is difficult to turn back contributions even if formal approval has not been obtained.

The main source of income for day-to-day expenses is the sale of services to the sick funds. Within the oversight of the Ministry of Health, the hospital – like other general hospitals – negotiates a capped annual budget with each sick fund, based on anticipated volume of service multiplied by the fees that are determined by the Ministry of Health. However, hospitals can offer discounts to sick funds in exchange for hospitals channelling patients to them. In the case of the hospital concerned, a process of active bargaining takes place, since in Jerusalem the sick funds face little resistance from patients told to go to the hospital. The situation can fluctuate from year to year, however, as the hospital's main competition in Jerusalem – a nearby medium-sized hospital – can also offer discounts to sick funds. To paraphrase the director of that hospital: the amount raised in contributions by the two hospitals is used each year to cover losses that occur when sick funds transfer volume from one hospital to the other. In addition to payments from the sick funds, which account for about 80% of the budget, the hospital receives revenue for childbirths (paid for separately by the National Insurance Institute), services provided to the military, and private payments.

Accountability framework

The hospital director is accountable to the Board of Directors, of which one third is representatives of the JWO. The hospital – since it is subsidized in part by government funding – must report its financial status to the Ministry of Health and the Ministry of Finance.

The Ministry of Health keeps track of hospital admissions, discharges, length of stay, and bed turnover, broken down by major departments. Quality measures, such as adherence to process guidelines, are collected by the Ministry in the context of a national effort to improve hospital care, but these data are not made public. In the past, casemix-adjusted measures of mortality from heart surgery were collected by the Ministry of Health, but when the data leaked to the press, physicians (on a nationwide basis) ceased cooperating with the monitoring effort. The hospital conducts patient satisfaction surveys that are used for internal purposes. There is a safety and quality improvement unit to monitor infections, medical error and adherence to safety measures within the hospital, the authority of which relies on the backing of the hospital Directorate.

Hospital mortality must be reported to the Ministry of Health, and in cases of suspected error or malfeasance, the Ministry may create an investigatory board, with the possibility of sanctions, such as loss of medical licence for a period of time for the specific staff involved. There are conflicting opinions over whether investigation by peers under the auspices of the Ministry of Health leads to severe enough sanctions in cases of medical error and accidents.

8.3.2 Operational governance issues

Limits on hospital strategy

The hospital does not face serious limitations from a political authority in terms of setting its overall goals and objectives, or expanding its activities.

Internal operational structure

The hospital is free to determine its own internal structure, but this is subject to the significant role played by department heads in the hospital hierarchy. Since the early 2000s, a number of hospital divisions, such as internal medicine, have been created, but department heads still are very powerful. Departmental budgets have been implemented in some cases, but these budgets do not include personnel costs, as these are determined by national staffing requirements and pay scales. The hospital retains some discretion in terms of allocating nurses across departments. The management can seek to improve coordination and communication, for example in the use of common resources such as pharmacy. However, the strength of department directors limits the degree to which changes in structure and behaviour at the departmental level can be managed by the hospital Directorate. The professional structure of the hospital is influenced primarily by the medical staff, again dominated by department heads.

Responsibility and decision-making capacity

Department heads have the lion's share of responsibility and decision-making capacity. Other actors, such as unions, elected officials and even the hospital Directorate have little say in the internal management of the departments. If a decision involves creating a new service, or purchasing new equipment with implications for the overall hospital budget, the hospital Directorate will be involved. But decisions that fall within the framework of a departmental budget – for example, to obtain certain pharmaceuticals or supplies through outsourcing – need not involve directors above the department level. Decisions such as whether to introduce experimental drugs not covered by the national health insurance are more or less made at the level of the individual physician, and there are no definitive directives from hospital management on this type of matter.

Monitoring and internal intelligence

The hospital monitors financial data relating to patient flows, as well as utilization of resources such as pharmaceuticals, laundry, and so on. The monitoring system is created by the hospital, over and above the minimal requirements to report to the Ministry of Health regarding admissions, discharges, length of stay and bed turnover, which are reported at the department level. The hospital has begun to monitor infections, adherence to practice guidelines, mortality and nosocomial infections at the department level. This monitoring is more or less on a voluntary basis, although the hospital has cooperated with Ministry of Health processes relating to quality assessment, with confidentiality maintained. The hospital has an electronic patient record system in place, which is accessible to any physician in the hospital who has the national identification number of the patient in question available. This system is internal and is not immediately able to be interfaced with external patient records, such as those maintained by the sick funds. These various databases can be used by the hospital Directorate to evaluate performance at the departmental level and to relate these measurements to hospital goals, although the latter – as already mentioned – are largely determined by the department heads.

Incentive schemes

Outside of private practice, there are few financial incentives that can be applied to medical, nursing and other staff. Performance of individual staff members is measureable, but rewards take the form of formal recognition, prizes, prestige and so on, rather than financial remuneration.

8.4 Case study 2: a large government-owned hospital in the Tel Aviv area

8.4.1 Strategic governance issues

Structural institutional framework

The hospital is required to provide certain basic services but has considerable latitude to provide additional services. The main difference with regard to additional services, relative to Case study 1 in the previous section, is that the government-owned hospital is prohibited from providing private services and offering choice of physicians in exchange for private payments. It is important to note that until 2004 this hospital had arrangements in place called "research funds", to which patients were "encouraged" to contribute by their specific physicians. This arrangement was declared illegal by the State Attorney General in 2004, and the question arose regarding whether this hospital should be permitted to have the type of private service arrangements that are permitted in the hospital discussed in Case study 1. This issue has not yet been resolved.

Much like Case study 1, the hospital concerned here is deeply involved in creating new services, which it does subject to Ministry of Health approval. If the changes do not involve new budgets or salaries, it is unlikely that the Ministry will intervene. Much like the hospital in Case study 1, initiatives of department directors lead to the creation of new services and institutes, along with the purchase of equipment. The Directorate is required to approve these initiatives, but if the business plan is sound, there is little reason to refuse.

Financial framework

Like the first hospital, the second is subject to staffing levels and salary scales determined in national negotiations between the Israel Medical Association, various unions, the Ministry of Health and the Ministry of Finance. This hospital also is very active in raising contributions for the creation of new services, physical expansion and the purchase of new equipment. It has "friends of" organizations in a number of countries that raise money for the hospital. Again, once earmarked contributions have been obtained, it is difficult for the Ministry of Health to intervene and refuse the hospital permission to use them.

This hospital is subject to the same reimbursement arrangements as the hospital in Case study 1 in terms of contracting with sick funds, up to an overall negotiated budgetary ceiling. The hospital agrees to discount arrangements with the sick funds, but also has aggressively responded to attempts by sick funds to transfer patients to other hospitals, by threatening to deny access to highly sophisticated treatments and publicly decrying the interference of the sick funds in the choice and treatment of the insured population.

Accountability framework

In most government-owned hospitals, there is no public Board of Trustees. However, this particular hospital is a leading innovator in the system, due to the charismatic leadership of its long-standing director. Thus, the hospital has appointed a Board of Directors of its own accord, but a question arises regarding how much control this board has over the operating managers. The hospital director is technically subordinate to the Director-General of the Ministry of Health, but is largely an independent agent, due to precedents set by an earlier, very entrepreneurial director, who still retains extensive influence in the hospital and the wider health system. At this point, it is important to mention that Directors-General of the Ministry of Health have often come from and returned to the post of director of a Ministry of Health hospital. This creates the perception of a conflict of interest, but perhaps highlights even more clearly the blurred boundaries and patterns of informal influence that exist within the system. The hospital reports to the two ministries the same basic patient flow data as the first hospital analysed, and the ministries retain data on its financial performance. The hospital participates on a voluntary basis in the various quality-improvement efforts being run by the Ministry of Health.

8.4.2 Operational governance issues

Limits on hospital strategy

Aside from providing certain core services, the hospital operates without significant intervention from the Ministry of Health and the Ministry of Finance, and is largely free to develop strategic initiatives aiming to provide new services, create new institutes, initiate physical expansion and purchase equipment, provided these do not impact on the hospital budget or require the provision of additional beds.

Internal operational structure

The hospital is free to determine its own internal structure – for example, whether to create a divisional structure – but, as in Case study 1, department heads are particularly powerful and so the department level remains the main subsystem within the formal structure. With the cooperation of the department heads, the hospital Directorate can reallocate personnel subject to national staffing requirements. The Directorate can also initiate communication and coordination arrangements and create the necessary information (and other) systems to enable this.

Responsibility and decision-making capacity

Decisions regarding allocation of resources, such as departmental budgets and use of central services (such as pharmacy, laundry, etc.) are made by the Directorate, with the cooperation of department heads. As in the first hospital, medical decisions remain largely in the hands of the treating physician, with little intervention by higher levels within the hospital hierarchy.

Monitoring and internal intelligence

Like the first hospital studied, this hospital has in place an electronic patient record system that enables tracking and coordination of patient care. The hospital monitors the financial and medical performance of the various departments.

Incentives

Without the incentive of private practice, the hospital has concerns about any external inducement – such as that provided by a new private hospital recently opened by one of the sick funds – to entice physicians to leave early in the day, or perhaps to change positions altogether, in order to perform private procedures elsewhere.

8.5 Case study 3: a large non-profit-making sick fund-owned hospital in the Tel Aviv area

This hospital operates much like the one in Case study 2, and is a major competitor with the latter. The main difference is that since it is, by ownership, part of a sick fund, its autonomy is influenced by the degree to which its strategies and tactics must conform to the goals of the organization that owns it. Moreover, as the sick fund is divided into regions, the hospital functions within the managerial sphere of influence at regional level. Since it is the flagship hospital of the sick fund, it is also directly linked to national-level management. In summary, the hospital appears to enjoy levels of autonomy similar to those of the hospital in Case study 2, since it can and does conclude service contracts with other sick funds (among other factors). The hospital has initiated many special services and institutes, such as a major children's hospital, funded to a great extent by revenue raised abroad.

8.5.1 Strategic governance issues

Structural institutional framework

This hospital is a tertiary medical centre required to provide the same range of services as the two hospitals already discussed in this chapter's previous case studies. It can expand its range of services subject to Ministry of Health approval and that of the national headquarters of the sick fund. Private services of any kind are prohibited. Installation and operation of new equipment is dependent on certificate of need approval.

Financial framework

The hospital's budget is based on the national capped prospective budget system. It has no revenue from private, fee-for-service care, but receives contributions from "friends" organizations and other philanthropic sources.

Accountability framework

The hospital reports to the national headquarters of the sick fund, as well as to the Ministry of Health. It has no separate Board of Directors.

8.5.2 Operational governance issues

Limits on hospital strategy

This hospital can initiate new services, but only subject to approval from the national sick fund headquarters and the Ministry of Health.

Internal operational structure

Shifting of resources or restructuring within the hospital are at the discretion of the hospital director, but if these represent significant changes involving hiring and firing, or require additional budgets, approval is required from the national sick fund headquarters.

Responsibility and decision-making capacity

The director of the hospital has the least autonomy of any of the directors discussed in this chapter. All decisions are subject to sick fund headquarters approval and to agreements with local unions. As in any hospital, much depends on the unique hospital culture and the informal relationship between the hospital director and the local union.

Monitoring and internal intelligence

The hospital director has access to data at the individual patient level, as well as to the data that are prepared for reporting to the Ministry of Health.

Incentives

The director of the hospital has no financial incentives to offer to encourage high-quality performance or extra work. (S)He can encourage, for example, individual department heads to pursue department-based initiatives, but implementation of projects involving finance and expansion outside of the budget must be approved by the national sick fund headquarters and the Ministry of Health.

8.6 Case study 4: a private hospital owned by one of the sick funds in the Tel Aviv area

This hospital is very different from the other cases. It can determine its own portfolio of services, and it emphasizes mostly elective surgery, subject to approval from the Ministry of Health. It appeals to those who have supplemental insurance (75% of the population). While some physicians (in particular new immigrant physicians) work solely for the hospital, it also relies on physicians who have been trained in the public sector, along with many who combine public and private work – the latter presumably "after hours", later in the afternoon and evening. The governance structure is that of a private corporation, but the role of the non-profit-making sick fund as an owner is not clear. The hospital is not intended to prioritize members of its umbrella sick fund as part of its strategy. It is also not clear how profits are allocated, especially between the hospital and the sick fund.

8.6.1 Strategic governance issues

Structural institutional framework

The hospital is governed by a Board of Directors, established with input from the sick fund's General Assembly. The Board has a financial subcommittee and an oversight subcommittee headed by a paid chairman. The governance structure of the hospital includes a medical chief of staff, a financial director, a director for operations and logistics, a director for human resources and a chief economist.

Financial framework

Large investments (such as in real estate) require approval of the Board, as do large purchases of equipment. Smaller investments can be made by the director at her/his discretion. The hospital has individual pricing agreements with the different sick funds, and tries not to favour the parent sick fund.

Accountability framework

The hospital is accountable to the Board and the shareholders, the latter being mainly the owner (that is, the sick fund).

8.6.2 Operational governance issues

Limits on hospital strategy

The hospital is subject to Ministry of Health approval for expansion of services, if this requires an increase in the number of beds. As Ministry of Health hospitals are in competition with private hospitals, this can create the perception of a conflict of interest.

Internal operational structure

The hospital has weekly meetings of its economic managers and of the hospital Directorate, in which the director plays the dominant role, and most of the director's decisions are approved by the Board.

Responsibility and decision-making capacity

The hospital can set its own prices and is not subject to tariffs set by the Ministry of Health. It pays its nursing staff according to national collective agreements, which serve as a benchmark even though this is not required. Hiring and firing of physicians is subject to national labour laws, and the hospital has an agreement with the National Labor Federation in this regard.

Monitoring and internal intelligence

The hospital has invested large sums in installing advanced IT, providing detailed information to the management. The data are used to provide financial reports to the Board and its oversight committees.

Incentives

The director has available a number of physician reimbursement arrangements. Some physicians work for a salary and can negotiate additional payments directly with patients. Other physicians work on a fee-for-service basis.

8.7 Discussion

When considering governance of hospitals in Israel, it is important to take into account a number of background factors, discussed here.

- Like many systems in Israel, the hospital sector is both pluralistic and centralized at the same time, due to the fact that many institutions began to function before the State of Israel was created in 1948, and thus resist the attempts of central government to exert control.

- Israeli political and managerial culture, in general, is characterized by blurred boundaries among sectors, as well as incompletely developed concepts and approaches regarding regulation and accountability. Israeli actors are caught between a naïve belief in technocratic planning and a cynical belief that in the end management is a matter of improvization and "hand-to-hand political combat".

- As with all systems, formal rules of ownership and regulation cannot capture all the nuances of the hospital environment and, in a country notable for "informal" arrangements of all kinds (Galnoor, 2007), this point is particularly relevant. Policy ideas, both imported and domestic, play an important role in understanding:

  - the hospital policy process;
  - the perceptions of key actors regarding the environment in which they are functioning;
  - the behaviour of key actors; and
  - the results of the system in terms of quality and cost.

Thus, although the Israeli case is very fluid, or perhaps due to this fluidity of circumstances, the Ministry of Health has been able to institutionalize quality measures within the hospitals. This involves, among other elements, a great deal of trust among the actors involved. Hospitals grant access to Ministry of Health staff, who observe and gather quality and performance data, with the cooperation of hospital staff. The data remain privileged information for the individual hospitals, but aggregate data are made available so that each hospital can assess its performance in the area of quality improvement. Such a cooperative – rather than coercive – approach may be an important element of governance in many health systems.

In terms of the approach to governance taken in this book, the Israeli case may or may not be a case of good (or at least workable) order, but one would be hard pressed to say that it reflects any clear governing body or set of rules. What we have is a patchwork of different frameworks, with a particularly peculiar combination of centralized control and autonomy.

From the centralized point of view, hospital staffing levels and pay scales are centrally controlled, based on negotiations among parties that do not include the hospitals per se. Representatives of the Israel Medical Association, individual labour unions, the Ministry of Health and the Ministry of Finance are parties to these negotiations and the hospitals are for the most part simply passive recipients of the results. Since about 70% of every hospital's budget is allocated to salaries, it is significant that this proportion of the budget is largely not controlled by the individual hospital directors and managers.

However, and perhaps ironically, due to the overlapping authorities implicit in these arrangements, there is little centralized control over hospital activity within the framework of the other 30% of their budgets. Hospitals use this smaller yet still significant proportion of their funding to carry out their own strategies, which usually involve developing new services, physical expansion initiatives and purchasing expensive equipment. Much of the 30% is raised through contributions for fixed assets, the use of which comes at the expense of operating budgets. So, instead of a unified, integrated method of allocating and spending resources, there are two main flows of funding, operating somewhat separately but each symbiotic with the other.

In the areas of quality of care, safety and information systems, the individual hospitals are mostly in control, but the Ministry of Health tries – and succeeds, to an extent – to introduce common measures and processes. While the hospitals are very much competitors – at least in the above-mentioned 30% of funding within the hospitals' sphere of influence – there seems to be some implicit interest in cooperating on quality improvement, as well as some potential for the creation of common and perhaps even linked data sets.

This raises the interesting question of whether governance (at least at the national level) should aim to create a unified, consistent, accountable structure for general hospitals. Perhaps more realistic – or even preferable – would be a more implicit balance based on a combination of centralized control and high levels of autonomy, which can constitute a healthy balance between a rigid form of national bureaucracy and an unfettered free market.

8.8 Conclusions

The case of hospital governance in Israel is perhaps best captured by putting it in the context of overall Israeli governance patterns which seem to combine a high degree of cynicism regarding formalism and rules, with strong input from the legal system, and increasing professionalism among planners, regulators and providers within the health system. Thus, the Israeli hospital – to varying degrees within different sectors – is at the same time highly constrained and also able to find "room to manoeuvre". It would seem reasonable to think that such an approach would be applicable in social services more broadly. However, the Israeli health system, with all of its problems, seems to have achieved a better form of governance that other sectors, such as education and welfare, at least as far as public perceptions of system performance are concerned. Perhaps it is the link to medical science that enables the system to coalesce around issues of quality and cost in a flexible form of governance that is perhaps a recipe to be considered for all health systems.

8.9 References

[Anonymous] (2004). *Lion Committee report on management of government-owned hospitals* (in Hebrew). Tel Aviv, Israeli Ministry of Health.

Bennun G, Berlowitz Y, Shani M (2005). *The health system in Israel.* Tel Hashomer, Sheba Medical Center Research Fund.

Chinitz D, Rosen B (1993). *A tale of two markets: hospital competition in Jerusalem and Tel Aviv.* Jerusalem, JDC-Brookdale Institute.

Feder-Bubis P (2006). *Perceptions of organizational change in Israeli hospitals* (in Hebrew) [PhD dissertation]. Jerusalem, Hebrew University.

Galnoor I (2007). *Public administration Israel.* Jerusalem, Hebrew University Academon Press.

Ministry of Health (2002). *Amorai Committee report on public medicine and the status of the physician* (in Hebrew). Tel Aviv, Israeli Ministry of Health.

Rosen B (2009). Israel: health system review. *Health Systems in Transition,* 11(2):1–226.

State of Israel (1940). *Public Health Ordinance.* Jerusalem, the Knesset.

State of Israel (2002). *Budget Fundamentals Law.* Jerusalem, the Knesset.

Chapter 9
Netherlands

Hans Maarse and Léon Lodewick

9.1 Introduction

This chapter investigates the structure of hospital governance in the Netherlands. Governance has been a much-used term in Dutch health care policy-making over the last decade (Meurs & Schraven, 2006). The term mostly refers to relations, tasks, formal competences and responsibilities of key players, in particular but not exclusively – one of the fundamental hypotheses of this book – the Executive Board and the Supervisory Board.

Hospital governance issues (for example, the role, size, appointment and remuneration of Executive Board and Supervisory Board members) has always been unregulated in the Netherlands. Fundamental changes are currently taking place in the hospitals' environment, triggering a need to reconsider governance structure and functioning. To fill the "regulatory gap", the representative associations of health care providers agreed in 2005 upon a self-regulatory "Health Care Governance Code", describing the structure of relations, tasks, competences and responsibilities of the Executive Board and Supervisory Board. However, the Code had no legal basis, as a consequence of which, formal enforcement mechanisms were lacking.

This chapter focuses on the governance of *general hospitals* but most of the content equally applies to other provider organizations, such as nursing homes, psychiatric hospitals or organizations providing ambulatory and/or residential care to specific categories of patients/clients. There are important differences, however, in particular regarding the role of the medical staff. Whereas a large proportion of specialist staff in general hospitals are self-employed and paid on a fee-for-service basis (as described in more detail later), medical staff in non-hospital provider organizations have employee status and are paid a salary. The governance of academic hospitals also differs in some respects from the governance of general hospitals – not only because of their teaching and research function, but also because of the government's competence to formally appoint the members of the hospitals' Supervisory Boards, usually on the recommendation of the Supervisory Board itself. Contrary to most general hospitals, all physicians in academic hospitals are salaried employees.

The structure of this chapter is as follows.

- Our analysis starts with a brief overview of the general structure of hospital care and a number of fundamental changes in its regulatory and socio-cultural environment, which – as we will see – have major repercussions for hospital governance.

- Next, we briefly analyse the structure and functioning of hospital governance at strategic and operational levels.

- The final section discusses some new issues in hospital governance.

9.2 The structure of hospital care in the Netherlands

For decades, the Netherlands has had a Bismarckian type of health care system.

Hospitals are private non-profit-making entities with the social purpose of providing specialist care to patients – that is, as private entities they do not form part of the state hierarchy. They were mainly founded by religious communities and municipal governments. Over time, however, all public hospitals were converted into non-profit-making private organizations, with the last wave of "privatization" occurring in the early 1990s. Until now, health regulation has always contained a ban on profit-making hospitals owned by private investors, but this is currently being reconsidered, and in the near future the ban may be replaced with a new regulation, termed "regulated returns on investment", as part of the ongoing market-oriented reform (Van de Ven & Schut, 2008).

An important characteristic of hospital care in the Netherlands is that most medical specialists (hereafter specialists) work in a hospital setting. Each hospital has outpatient departments for specialists to treat patients. The number of specialists working full time or part time in private practice has always been fairly low, although there are indications that the situation is currently altering somewhat, due to the rapid growth of the market in ITCs (*zelfstandige behandelcentra*). The number of general hospitals has dropped from about 200 in 1950 to 95 in 2009, including eight academic hospitals and two specialized hospitals (Nederlandse Zorgautoriteit, 2009). The decline was mainly the result of regional mergers to improve the quality of care (better conditions for 24-hour continuity of care, more room for subspecialties) and/or survival financially. Merger hospitals also hoped to reinforce their market position by achieving some economies of scale and scope. Due to consolidations, the average number of beds per general hospital significantly increased from 349 in 1980 to 498 in 2008 (in 2008 the smallest hospitals had 138 beds and the largest had 1368 beds). This increase was paralleled with a fall in the total number of general hospital beds from about 60 000 beds in 1980 to approximately 42 350 beds in 2008.

Although the general trend in hospital care for the last half century has been one of concentration, currently there is a trend towards some deconcentration, in particular in the field of elective care (Maarse & Normand, 2009). The number of ITCs has spectacularly increased from 30 centres in the year 2000 to approximately 200 by the end of 2009. This growth was triggered by the waiting list crisis in the late 1990s, as well as calls for entrepreneurship and market competition in hospital care. The government also made it easier for new provider organizations to enter the market. ITCs are currently mainly active in routine elective (planned) services in various fields, including ophthalmology, dermatology, orthopaedic surgery, cosmetic surgery, radiology, cardiology and maternity and child care (obstetrics). Although the number of new entrants looks spectacular, the volume of care they deliver is still only a small fraction of total hospital care.

The Health Insurance Act (*Zorgverzekeringswet*) – which (as part of the market-oriented reform) came into force in 2006 and integrated the former Sickness Fund Scheme and private health insurance into a universal mandatory scheme – covers, among others, hospital care, GP care, outpatient prescription drugs and many other services. The Act is implemented by health insurers, which may function as profit-making insurers. Subscribers pay a government-set income-related contribution, plus – to foster competition – an insurer-set nominal fee (flat-rate premium). The government also determines the benefits package. Consumers are free to choose their insurer and are permitted to switch once a year. Insurers are obliged to accept each applicant. The Exceptional Medical Expenses Scheme (*Algemene Wet Bijzondere Ziektekosten*) mainly covers long-term care, such as residential care in a nursing home or care for people who have mental disabilities. It is a universal and mandatory scheme that is financed by means of an income-related contribution.

A key element of the ongoing market-oriented reform (Helderman et al., 2005) with potentially considerable consequences for hospitals is the upgrading of the role of insurers. Hospitals and insurers may now sign a contract on the price of medical services. Insurers also show greater interest in the quality of hospital care. If an insurer concludes that quality is substandard in a hospital, it may decide not to contract that hospital. A good example of this is the announcement of an insurer in 2010 that it would no longer contract four hospitals for breast cancer surgery, because these hospitals did not meet volume standards and patient satisfaction was considered to be less than satisfactory. Not surprisingly, the insurer's decision aroused great public attention. Nevertheless, since then, more insurers have announced their intention to opt for selective contracting and no longer to contract hospitals which do not meet volume standards and/or other quality standards (Maarse & Paulus, 2011).

Such changes in the regulatory and social environment have made most hospitals more vulnerable than in the past. The present strategic governance agenda is "densely populated" with issues such as the portfolio of medical services, appointment of new specialists, (weak) financial position requiring deep expenditure cuts, quality of care and patient safety, financing of (re)construction plans and other capital investments, IT, human resources, the establishment of new departments, implementing process innovations to make hospital care more patient friendly, revising the general structure of hospital governance, consolidations and property-related issues, and so on. The underlying purpose is to consider how to deliver efficient, innovative and demand-driven health care of high quality to patients. Other strategic issues include the relationship between the Executive Board and medical staff, the employees' council, insurers, financial agents and (last but not least) the general public. The call for greater public accountability has become ever louder over the last decade, making hospitals no longer a closed bastion and rather insensitive to the opinion of referring doctors (in particular GPs) and patients. Strategic hospital governance is now much more complicated than it has probably ever been.

9.3 Strategic hospital governance

This section gives a brief overview of hospital governance in the Netherlands. It addresses first the strategic dimension of governance, with subsections on institutional arrangements (the tasks, responsibilities and functioning of the major players in hospital governance: the Supervisory Board, the Executive Board, the Board of Medical Specialists and even the role of employees and clients), followed by the financial and accountability arrangements linked to the private non-profit-making status of the country's hospitals. Finally, it addresses the operational aspects of hospital governance.

9.3.1 Institutional arrangements

Almost all hospitals have the legal structure of a foundation (*stichting*). Neither the Minister of Health, Welfare and Sport (hereafter Minister of Health) nor local public authorities are involved in the appointment of the hospital's Executive Board and Supervisory Board members (the arrangement is different for academic centres). As a non-profit-making entity, hospitals cannot (yet) be owned by agents with a commercial purpose.

The foundation possesses the government's licence to provide inpatient and outpatient care and may establish private limited companies (*besloten vennootschap*) as the legal vehicle for health care delivery. The corporation usually holds 100% of the shares of these companies, although a lower percentage (still usually over 50%) is also possible. In the latter case, specialists may act as co-shareholders.

As private non-profit-making entities, hospitals belong to what is usually termed the private initiative sector (*particulier initiatief*), which co-exists with the government sector, the market sector and the informal sector. Organizations in this sector are actively involved in the provision of publicly funded services. This model is used not only in health care but also in many other sectors of public policy (such as education, welfare, housing, etc.). It rests upon the principle of subsidiarity in public policy-making, according to which the state should "delegate" the provision of public services as much as possible to private initiative.

The hospital's legal structure is increasingly viewed as a strategic governance issue because of the market-oriented reform and the call for greater entrepreneurship in hospital care. However, it is as yet unclear how the legal structure of hospitals will evolve. Recently, the government announced new legislation obligating hospitals to adopt a so-called "social enterprise" structure, which can be described as a private but publicly funded service delivery organization, the purpose of which is not to make (or maximize) profit but rather to provide efficient and high-quality services to its clients. The legislative proposal will be briefly discussed in the section 9.5.

Supervisory Board

Each hospital has a Supervisory Board (*Raad van Toezicht*), performing the following functions:

- appointment and discharge of the members of the hospital Executive Board;

- supervision of the functioning of the Executive Board and its individual members;

- appointment and discharge of the external accountant;

- approval of specific decisions and documents of the Executive Board, including the annual budget estimate, annual accounts and annual report, strategic and investment plans, decisions relating to property transactions and decisions on consolidations; and

- remuneration of the Executive Board members, and functioning as a sounding board for the hospital Executive Board.

There are no formal rules regarding the number of members of the Supervisory Board, which in practice varies between 5 and 11. The board composition is based on cooptation. The Board appoints its own chairman and members, with no role for the Minister of Health or local politicians. For a long period, board members were not selected because of their expertise but for their position in the upper echelons of the local community. For about a decade, however, there has been a trend towards professionalizing the composition of the Supervisory Board. Increasingly, boards select their members because of their assumed expertise. Another objective is to have a variety of expertise "on board".

Following the Health Care Governance Code, appointments as member of the Supervisory Board are for four years. Each member can only be reappointed once (but this may vary). Members are paid a fee by the hospital ranging from €4000 to €15 000 a year. There are usually about six board meetings a year, but the chairman usually meets the members of the Executive Board on a more regular basis.

The Supervisory Board is not in charge of hospital management, which is the exclusive responsibility of the Executive Board. Supervision requires that it operates at distance from the Executive Board. There is no clear answer regarding what operating "at distance" means. Supervision is a subtle matter, requiring much expertise and a sensitive antenna. It is also a matter of trust in the Executive Board, but that trust should be permanently deserved.

There are signs that Supervisory Boards often do not function well (Lodewick, 2008). It frequently happens that the board members are not well informed regarding the real issues that the hospital faces and do not know "what is really going on in their hospital". A crisis is regularly a surprise to the Supervisory Board. This may be due to the fact that its members lack the expertise to supervise effectively, lack sufficient time to perform their work properly or tend to function at too great a distance to be effective. The Supervisory Board's dependence on information from the Executive Board (incomplete, outdated or filtered) may be another problem, although the Supervisory Board may also receive signals from medical staff or the employees' council, among others (this mostly happens in crisis situations). A more recent development is that Supervisory Boards are criticized by politicians after financial problems or problems in the quality of hospital care have become public. These problems tend to lead to difficult questions being asked about the role and expertise of the Supervisory Board, often accompanied by a call for regulatory government measures.

A structural issue relating to the Supervisory Board model in Dutch hospital care concerns to whom the Board is responsible. Hospitals are not owned by public authorities, private investors or other private organizations (such as a religious organization), but rather by a foundation without members or shareholders. So the question is, who supervises the supervisor? In the past this question did not play a significant role but the situation has now changed, for at least two reasons. First, ongoing changes in the hospitals' regulatory and sociocultural environment have made hospital governance much more complicated. Hospitals with poor performance can easily and quickly run into considerable trouble. As a consequence, the role of the Supervisory Board has gained importance. Second, hospitals nowadays function simultaneously in the public and private sectors. They are viewed as non-profit-making entities exposed to the laws of competition (market organization), but at the same time as agencies performing a public function funded by "public" resources (task organization).

This hybrid status has important implications, as illustrated by the thorny political issue of remunerating the members of the Executive Board. Politicians accuse supervisory boards of being too generous. Many consider the salary of the Prime Minister (about €180 000) to be a maximum level of remuneration, but recent research (Tulleneers, 2010) found that, in 2008, income of members of hospital Executive Boards averaged at €158 000, with a ceiling of €266 000 (excluding bonuses). A total of 44% of the executives exceeded the standard income. Furthermore, average income for academic hospitals executives was €219 000, with a top ceiling of €283 000 (before bonuses). The government is currently undertaking initiatives to curb the remuneration of such Executive Boards. There is now also regulation to hold individual Supervisory Board members liable in case of manifest financial failure. Media attention to remuneration issues has also significantly increased since 2005, when hospitals were obligated to publish detailed information on the yearly payments to each member of the Executive Board and Supervisory Board in their financial accounts.

Supervisory Boards have reacted to these developments by seeking to improve the professionalism of their work. As already indicated, their members are increasingly selected on the basis of expertise, and advertising the recruitment of new members has become common practice. Of specific importance in this respect is the variety of expertise needed on the Board. Furthermore, the Netherlands Association of Health Care Supervisors (*Nederlandse Vereniging van Toezichthouders in de Zorg*) organizes various activities to professionalize the role of Supervisory Boards and has also undertaken an initiative to revise the Health Care Governance Code (see section 9.5).

Executive Board

The Executive Board (*Raad van Bestuur*) is a relatively new actor in hospital governance. Until the early 1980s many hospitals had a medical superintendent (*geneesheer-directeur*) who combined – usually on a 50/50 basis – her/his medical practice with the hospital directorship. In that position (s)he was supported by the directors for nursing and financial affairs. Currently, each hospital has an Executive Board of between one and three members. There is no compulsory requirement that a person with a medical background should be a member of the Board; members are increasingly recruited from outside the medical profession, reflecting the concept that hospitals must be run like an enterprise. As already mentioned, the Executive Board members are appointed by the Supervisory Board, although the employees' council and the clients' council (see the following subsections) have acquired the legal right to give their opinion on each appointment. Usually, the Medical Staff Board (*Bestuur Medische Staf* (BMS)) is also involved in the appointment procedure and asked for its opinion.

The Executive Board is empowered to define the institutional structure of the hospital, including the set-up of clinical and other subunits, as well as internal accountability relationships. It is also in charge of the hospital's financial policy, investment plans and relations with financing agents (banks), the medical service portfolio of the hospital and issues relating to quality of care. It is held accountable for the strategic and operational governance of the hospital in its entirety, as well as for the hospital's relationships with the "outside world" (Minister of Health, other provider organizations, health insurers, financial agents/banks and – last but not least – the media).

In theory, the Executive Board can make unilateral decisions, but in practice this does not work well. To be successful, it must continuously build a sufficient level of support for its decisions within the organization. For a set of specific decisions, it even needs the formal approval of the medical staff and the employees' council. The decisions for which formal approval of the medical staff is required are formulated in the Medical Staff Document (*Document Medische Staf*). This document was given legal basis by the Integration Act (2000), which "defined" the hospital as an integrated medical specialist enterprise (*geïntegreerd medisch-specialistisch bedrijf)*. In short, the Executive Board is in charge of most hospital governance matters (Lodewick, 2008).

Medical staff

Hospital governance cannot be fully understood without taking the role of the medical staff into account. To understand their prominent role in hospital governance, it is important to make a distinction between two categories of specialists.

- About 30% of the specialists work in the Netherlands as hospital employees; they have an employee contract, are paid a salary and have a formal hierarchical relationship with the Executive Board.

- Specialists in the second category (about 70%) are self-employed. They work as quasi-entrepreneurs ("entrepreneur with tenure") in the hospital and are paid on a fee-for-service basis. Usually, they pay the hospital only for administrative and managerial support, but not for the use of medical facilities (as was the case until the early 1970s).

Whether specialists are employed or self-employed depends upon historical factors and local conditions. Generally speaking, paediatricians, rheumatologists, psychiatrists and to some extent neurologists are employed – as is the case with most support specialties (e.g. pharmacy, pathology, clinical physics, nuclear medicine). Radiologists are a clear exception: almost all of them are self-employed.

Self-employed medical specialists need a formal admission contract (*toelatingsovereenkomst*) with the hospital, granting them the right to provide inpatient and outpatient medical care in the hospital. The contract obligates the hospital to provide specialists with all facilities "according to the latest standards of medical science". It also contains obligations for specialists, for instance that they are required to follow the instructions of the Executive Board, to inform the Executive Board on medical errors and accidents, as well as "malfunctioning" colleagues. However, there may be a gap between the formal rules of the contract and what happens in reality.

Self-employed specialists are organized in specialist partnerships (*maatschappen*) and salaried specialists work in specialist departments (*vakgroepen*); there are no combinations of partnership and department (it is either one or the other). Their respective size varies according to specialty and type of hospital.

In many hospitals, employed and self-employed specialists are organized in the association of medical specialists (*Vereniging van Medisch Specialisten*), which every four years elects the members of the BMS. This Board frequently interacts with the Executive Board on strategic and operational issues, but most of the time it does so without a general mandate of the medical staff. As a consequence, the BMS must consult its constituency for approval of its agreements (or disagreements) with the Executive Board (Lodewick, 2008). The Executive Board considers the BMS to be a very important player in hospital governance and for that reason frequently consults with it. In fact, the Executive Board needs BMS support for all strategic decisions. To function properly, the "dual governance model" requires a BMS to hold a strong position in terms of the medical staff, and to be capable of achieving despite the opposition of specialist groups or individual specialists.

There is considerable variation in how the medical staff function in a hospital. Yet, a few general observations can be made. An initial observation is that most specialists have a strong orientation towards their own specialty/specialist group. As such, they often tend to act as a closed group, even if they know that one or more of their associates is malfunctioning in terms of medical care. Breaking the group code of silence is not appreciated. Each specialist group is primarily interested in its own affairs; the interests of the entire hospital are (at best) a secondary consideration. Specialists also underline their professional autonomy in medical care. The notion of professional accountability is still underdeveloped. Their emphasis upon professional autonomy may be so strong that specialists may adopt a hostile attitude towards any interference (as they see it) from hospital management in their affairs, even in those affairs for which hospital management is directly responsible. Specialist groups often lack a sufficient level of self-reflexivity and self-purifying capacity (Lodewick, 2008).

The relationship between the Executive Board and the medical staff can probably be best described as a mutual love/hate relationship. Specialists "love" the Board because it provides them with the facilities they need to care for patients, but they also "hate" it because they feel constrained in terms of their autonomy and must comply with a variety of bureaucratic procedures. Furthermore, it may require a lot of effort to achieve anything. The Executive Board, for its part, "loves" its medical specialists because of their expertise and commitment to patients (although some may misbehave!) and the willingness of many of them to participate in management affairs. However, it also often "hates" specialists because of their lack of cooperation in hospital programmes to encourage better performance, their egos and frequent lack of respect for their colleagues, their propensity towards conflict behaviour and their readiness to unite in order to impede top-level management – in particular, the members of the Executive Board in the event that they lose their confidence. It is evident that these tumultuous relationships usually have a strong impact on hospital governance (Lodewick, 2008).

Employees and clients

The Executive Board, the Board of Medical Specialists and the Supervisory Board are the most important – but not the only – internal players in hospital governance. Two other internal players include the employees' council (*ondernemingsraad*) and the client council (*cliëntenraad*).

The Law on Employees Council (*Wet op de Ondernemingsraad*) regulates for which decisions the council has the right of advice and the right of approval, respectively. If the council formally withholds its approval, the Executive Board may ask the court to annul the council's decision, but it cannot implement its decision during this procedure. The council can, therefore, be considered an important actor for the Executive Board, because it is the formal representative body of hospital employees.

In practice it often functions as a channel for the unions to influence hospital governance, particularly regarding decisions with direct impact on employees. It is wise to build up a relationship of trust with the council and to involve it in policy development at an early stage – not only to inform it but also to ask for its advice and to build a support network. Many Executive Boards meet regularly with the employees' council (although some tend to see it more as an obstacle in hospital governance than as crucial actor).

Hospitals are also obligated by law (*Wet Medezeggenschap Cliënten Zorginstellingen*) to have a client council (*cliëntenraad*) representing patients' interests in hospital governance. The role of the client council in governance should not be overstated in the case of acute hospitals, but is usually quite different for organizations providing long-term care. Here, patients/clients or their representatives (for example, parents or other family members) may play an active role.

9.3.2 Financial arrangements

Hospital funding is a crucial element of the Dutch hospitals' regulatory environment. Until 2005, hospitals were funded by a system of fixed budgets (introduced in the early 1980s), with three main components: an availability component, a capacity component and a production component. The latter was based upon yearly volume contracts between each hospital and insurers, and on the number of admissions, inpatient days, first outpatient visits and day care/surgery. The budgeting system had several flaws, the most serious of which probably was that it did not contain powerful incentives to perform better. Better performance was hardly rewarded, and poor performance hardly punished (Maarse, 1995).

As indicated, the relationships between the Executive Board and the medical staff are inherently tense, partly for financing reasons. The professional administrator will keep her/his power only as long as the medical staff perceive that their interests are being served effectively. This will be relatively easy if the interests of the specialists run parallel to those of the hospital's Board. However, their interests are often not (or only partly) aligned. Whereas specialists call for the latest technology and more support staff or space (beds), the Board is confronted with limited resources and must avoid deficits. The former model of fixed hospital budgets even created a fundamental conflict of interest between the Executive Board and self-employed specialists. Whereas specialists had an interest in producing a high volume of services to increase their private revenues, hospital management had a strategic interest in cost control because of the introduction of a fixed budget for materials, medicines, nursing staff, equipment, and so on.

To make hospital funding more performance related, a new casemix-based funding model was introduced in 2005. Hospitals are now paid a fixed sum of money for each of their 30 000 diagnosis–treatment combinations (DTCs), which can best be regarded as a kind of DRG for both inpatient and outpatient care. This number is scheduled to be reduced to about 3000 in 2012, as there is wide consensus that the current system is too complicated to function properly.

DTCs are also used as a tool for price competition. In 2006, about 10% of hospital production (by value) was funded on the basis of DTC prices negotiated between a hospital and each insurer (price per hospital and insurer may differ). Examples of free-price hospital care included cataracts, inguinal hernia, total hip replacement and diabetes care. The scope for price competition was extended to 20% in 2008 and 33% in 2009. There is uncertainty as yet regarding the ultimate scope of price competition, but there are reasons to assume that it will be substantially raised (possibly to some 70%). The prices of the DTCs that are not open to price negotiation are regulated by the Dutch Healthcare Authority (*Nederlandse Zorgautoriteit*).

As part of the current reform, the traditional central planning model has been replaced with a new model, affording hospitals much more autonomy for planning and investing in (re)construction. Market competition and entrepreneurship require hospitals to make their own strategic decisions regarding capacity and major investments (Maarse & Normand, 2009). The new model defines the responsibility of the Minister of Health in terms of a "system responsibility" or "responsibility for the continuity of care". The Minister no longer bears the responsibility for the continuity of an individual hospital or other provider organization.

The current reform also includes a significant revision of *capital investment financing*. Under the previous system, the costs of rent and depreciation of state-approved investments in construction works were financed by a retrospective mark-up on the per diem rate over a 40-year period, so that neither hospitals nor banks granting the loan incurred any financial risk. Under the new arrangement, hospitals will receive a prospective (normative) mark-up on the DTCs to finance capital investments, making the scope for capital investments contingent on the volume of services delivered. This is assumed to have important implications for strategic governance, making hospitals more aware of the costs of capital investments, in particular as regards their (re)construction plans. This assumption seems to be correct, now that hospitals have begun to reconsider their former "majeure" investment plans.

Another important implication is that the financing of a new hospital has become risk bound, not only for the hospital itself but also for the banks granting the loan – which, not surprisingly, have become insistent on seeing solid business plans. They may also require extra guarantees, for instance concerning the hospitals' financial performance. The new model may also attract private investor agencies in search for new investment opportunities, but they will only be interested if they expect a fair return on investment. Lifting or mitigating the ban on profit-making hospital care is seen as an effective instrument to attract private capital in the (re)construction of hospitals.

There are indications that the various changes in the hospital funding model – shifting from budgets to case-based payment by means of DTCs – have attenuated the fundamental conflict between the hospital management and clinicians, but there is no reason to believe that this will fully resolve the conflict.

9.3.3 Accountability arrangements

Significant changes have occurred in the hospital governance regulatory environment, as detailed in the subsections that follow.

Public accountability

The first significant change concerns the growing emphasis upon public accountability. Hospitals must now publish an annual financial account as well as an annual quality of care account.

A further notable development concerns the Health Care Inspectorate, which has become much more activist in its approach than it had been in the past. The attention of the media to problems in the hospital care setting – in particular serious medical errors and financial scandals – has also significantly increased over the last decade.

Important changes can also be observed in the hospital–patient relationship. A growing number of patients are becoming assertive. Patients also increasingly use Internet services to acquire information on the reputation and waiting times of hospitals or the treatment they must undergo. There are various web sites available to the public giving access to "objective and standardized" information on hospital performance; these sites also increasingly contain information on clinical outcomes (in 2010, hospitals were requested to disclose their standardized mortality rates). The purpose of publicizing information on hospital performance is to enable patients to make informed choices regarding their medical care. Public information is also expected to encourage hospitals to perform better.

Hospital–government relationship

As already pointed out, Dutch hospitals function relatively independent from politics, and politicians do not directly interfere in hospital governance. Apart from exceptional situations (such as huge financial problems), neither the Minister of Health nor local public authorities have any formal voice in the appointment of general hospitals' Executive Board and Supervisory Board members. However, regular bilateral contacts exist between the hospital and national and local governments.

Nevertheless, it is important to note in this regard that hospitals' contacts with the Ministry of Health have undergone significant changes over the last decade. Under the former centralist planning model, there was frequent contact relating to capacity issues. Hospitals needed the Ministry's approval on number of beds, specialist units and financial resources for building a new hospital or for implementing major reconstructive works. The approval procedure often entailed time-consuming consultations before a formal decision was made. Under the new regulation, the involvement of the Minister of Health has become much less intense because of the government's current policy to make hospitals largely responsible for their own investments. A few areas remain in which the Minister of Health is still directly involved in the planning of facilities, in particular concerning top-level clinical health services (transplantation surgery, top-level clinical interventions in paediatric care, including heart surgery and neonatology, stem-cell transplantation) and health services with major ethical implications (in vitro fertilization (IVF), clinical genetic research and advice).

Despite the government's policy to hold hospitals responsible for their own investments, financial problems and other affairs, the Minister of Health has recently become directly involved in some cases. A good example is the case of the *IJsselmeerziekenhuizen*, a hospital technically bankrupt by the end of 2008. The Minister stated that he was only responsible for the continuity of hospital care in the region in which the hospital was located. Yet, he eventually came to the conclusion that such bankruptcy would have an unacceptable disruptive effect upon the continuity of hospital care across the region. He decided accordingly to support the hospital financially and to appoint (together with the local and regional public authorities) one member of the newly formed Supervisory Board as a representative with veto power in all decisions with major financial implications (e.g. investments of €1 million or more). This case effectively illustrates the gap that may exist between the rhetoric of decentralization and market governance on the one hand and the "real world" of hospital governance on the other (Maarse & Paulus, 2011).

Interestingly, a trend towards more government regulation of health care governance can be observed at present. The government has come under increasing political pressure to restrain the remuneration of the Executive Board. Another example of this is the government's initiative to make the Supervisory Board members personally liable in case of manifest failure. Furthermore, as already mentioned, it has proposed regulation on a new legal structure for hospitals; following this proposal, hospitals should be converted into what is termed "a social enterprise" (*maatschappelijke onderneming*). As yet, however, the government has abstained from regulatory measures to enable the hospital sector to effectively self-regulate in terms of remuneration issues.

9.4 Operational hospital governance

The previous sections discussed various issues touching directly or indirectly upon strategic hospital governance. The complexity of strategic hospital governance requires the Executive Board to have significant personal and management skills in order to give direction to strategic matters. Strategic governance requires a great deal of steering and diplomatic capacity; it would be erroneous to see the Board as the top of a hierarchical organization in charge of making decisions and imposing instructions. Building support and mutual trust by effective communication is essential. In this respect, the Executive Board also fulfils a coaching role and an exemplary role. Experience shows that too much emphasis upon a hierarchical approach or behaviour is ultimately a ticket to failure. A complicating factor in this respect in the case of Netherlands is the frequent inability of the BMS to maintain unity within its ranks and to speak with one voice.

Any clear-cut dividing line between strategic and operational hospital governance is illusory because such a line in many ways simply does not exist. Both types of governance are tightly interwoven: strategic governance has important consequences for operational management and vice versa. The success of strategic management also depends to a great extent on the effectiveness and efficiency of operational governance. This section focuses its analysis on the internal organization of hospitals and the Executive Board's management of it.

Each hospital consists of a number of divisions (*divisies*) in which patient care is organized. Each division has its own budget and a manager in charge of the running of the division, directly reporting to the Executive Board. The manager is given a high degree of discretionary scope to manage her/his unit and is also made accountable for the performance of the division in its entirety (performance management). The manager is also a member of the management team of the hospital. Divisions usually encompass a number of subdivisions directed by unit managers (*afdelingshoofd*). In particularly large hospitals, the subdivision may not be the lowest level in the division structure.

An important development in operational governance concerns the introduction of dual management. Divisions and (often) subdivisions are managed by a duo comprising a full-time general manager and a part-time medical manager (0.1 or 0.2 full-time equivalents). This development reflects the need for optimal coordination of medical matters with other fields, including organizational, financial, logistic and personnel considerations.

Some hospitals have created a separate facilitative enterprise to organize their staff departments (human resources, finance, IT and so on). The managers of these departments are appointed by the Executive Board and are also directly responsible to it for the management of their department. The purpose of staff departments is to support and monitor the processes and performance of the divisions, and to advise the Executive Board.

The relationship between staff departments and divisions may be strained. Division managers often complain about the lack of support they receive from staff departments. Another complaint is that staff departments interfere in their internal affairs. A frequent complaint of staff managers concerns the reluctance of division managers to follow the general instructions and procedures set out by the Executive Board and staff departments for the proper functioning of the hospital.

9.5 New directions in hospital governance

In summary, hospitals in the Netherlands are private non-profit-making organizations, run by an Executive Board which is controlled by a Supervisory Board. With a few exceptions, there is no political involvement of the government or local public authorities in the appointment of the members of both boards.

As part of the ongoing market-oriented reform, the government's policy is to increase the autonomy of hospitals. The central planning of each hospital's capacity by the Minister of Health has been largely abolished, making hospitals responsible for their own investment plans. The transition from a fixed budget model to a new casemix-based funding model has made hospital funding considerably more performance related than it has been in the past. It is the government's policy to further increase the responsibility of hospitals for their own finances, but it remains to be seen how this plays out in the "real world", for instance, if the continuity of care in a region is at risk due to the bankruptcy of a large hospital.

Another challenge relates to the public accountability of hospitals. In the past, it was customary to assume that all hospitals performed well and that there was no reason for concern about the quality of hospital care. At present, hospital performance is increasingly measured by means of performance indicators. A growing body of information on structure, process and outcomes is made available to the public in order to encourage them to make informed decisions. Information on the remuneration of each member of the Executive and Supervisory Boards must also be disclosed to the public.

Furthermore, the hospital–insurer relationship is undergoing fundamental changes. The influence of insurers on hospital affairs is increasing, since insurers are no longer obligated to contract every hospital and may decide (as already briefly mentioned) not to contract a hospital because they consider the quality of specific medical services to be below standard or because hospital prices are not considered to be competitive. Contracting may have a significant impact on patient flows and for that reason gains strategic importance for hospital management. A related development with a similar effect is that insurers are tending to become increasingly more involved in the restructuring of the supply of hospital care, for instance by arguing that there are too many hospitals in a given region or that certain medical services must be concentrated in only a few hospitals for efficiency and quality of care reasons.

These developments have made hospital governance ever more complex. As a consequence, there is a call for a (further) professionalization of the Executive and Supervisory Boards. This explains the increasing prominence of the governance issue in Dutch hospital care. In the remainder of this section a few new developments in hospital governance are briefly discussed.

The first development concerns the position of medical specialists in hospital governance; they are involved in many ways. The Board of Medical Specialists is in frequent contact with the Executive Board regarding strategic and operational issues. Furthermore, the Executive Board has contact with many other individual or groups of specialists. Despite this contact, it is becoming increasingly evident that specialists could carry greater direct responsibility in terms of hospital management. In particular, many believe that they should be made responsible for the financial management of their unit. By means of a residual claim arrangement, they should have a financial interest in running their "business" properly. The basic idea underpinning this governance model is to optimally align the interests of the Executive Board and the directors of divisions with those of the specialists; all parties involved should have an interest in delivering efficient, state-of-the art, high-quality medical care. Creating distinct units with the hospital for delivering care to patients – with the co-responsibility of specialists for management – is an essential part of the new governance model.

Our second observation also concerns the role of specialists in hospital governance. Key elements in our analysis included their strong insistence on professional autonomy, their often hostile attitude towards hospital management, and the still existing culture of the "conspiracy of silence" in case of medical errors. There are indications that some changes are under way. There is a rising conscience in medical communities that specialists should assume greater responsibility for all that they do, including becoming more self-critical and setting up effective systems for personal performance evaluation. Frequent reports in the media also encourage specialists to look for constant improvement and to avoid errors. An open internal climate in which it becomes common to discuss failures is essential in this respect. The often difficult intervention of the Health Care Inspectorate in case of "malfunctioning" personnel is another important factor. These interventions do not only have negative repercussions for the hospital's reputation, but may also have far-reaching consequences for the specialists' own practice (for example, closure of surgery theatres affects many specialists).

The next development regards the Health Care Governance Code. This Code – a product of self-regulation – was agreed upon by the representative associations of health care provider organizations. Its immediate intention was to fill in the "regulatory gap" in health care governance, making any government regulation of it superfluous. The Code's ultimate intention was to professionalize governance and to generate a uniform model describing the structure of relations, tasks, competences and accountability of the Executive Supervisory Boards. The Code is currently being revised. It is a revision "under the shadow of hierarchy", because the provider associations are afraid that the government will take the lead in the reconstruction of health care governance. The changes in the new Code are not radical, however. As explained, the health care provider organizations are conceptualized as "social enterprises". The new aspect is that the Code applies not only to non-profit-making organizations but also to profit-making ones.

To avoid perpetuating a situation in which profit is a motive for performance, the Code defines profit as an "instrument", not as a goal in itself; returns on investments should take place in the context of the social purpose and accountability of the organization. The ambiguity of this regulation is evident. Another new element in the Code concerns the introduction of a "whistleblower" arrangement, giving employees or other stakeholders the right to inform the Executive Board of alleged irregularities of a general, operational or financial nature. The Executive Board is obligated to report on this to the chairman of the Supervisory Board. Finally, the Code is intended to avoid public regulation of the remuneration of the Executive Board. Remuneration must be in accordance with the social purpose of the provider organization; it must be fair and competitive but not excessive. This principle has been translated in concrete remuneration standards to take the size and complexity of the organization into consideration.

To what extent the associations' initiative to modernize the Code will be effective is yet to be seen. Against the background of lasting social and political discontent regarding the remuneration of the executives of private yet publicly funded service delivery organizations, such as hospitals, the government has announced public regulation on remuneration. The government's initiative highlights an interesting paradox; hospitals have a long tradition of great discretion in remunerating executives. The market-oriented reform aims to extend the decision rights of hospitals in order to ensure they are prepared for the new challenges of the market. At the same time, however, the hospitals' freedom in the remuneration of its executives is restricted by means of standards and other regulations (for example, no "golden handshake" after discharge). The new regulation somehow mirrors the politicians' distrust of the consequences of market competition.

A fourth development concerns the government's initiative to reinforce the position of the Executive Board relative to that of medical specialists. In the government's view, the position of the Board is rather weak, since it lacks effective instruments to hold specialists accountable for their actions. Specialists will be obligated to inform the Executive Board of the findings of external assessment commissions (currently, such an obligation does not exist).

Finally, it is important to note that when the government sent a regulatory proposal to the parliament in 2009, it described "social enterprise" in the introductory section as a private and publicly funded service delivery organization, the purpose of which is not to make (or maximize) profit, but to deliver efficient and high-quality services to its clients. The proposal is intended to ensure hospitals are ready for the entrepreneurial role they are ascribed in a model of regulated competition. A key issue in the proposal is the accountability problem; hospitals are owned by a foundation but it remains unclear to whom the foundation is accountable and who supervises the Supervisory Board.

The solution is sought in reinforcing the mutual relationship between service delivery organization and society. This is achieved through the introduction of a new voice arrangement: service delivery organizations are required to have a body representing the interests of the stakeholders. The stakeholder body is given the legal right to be consulted periodically, to be asked for its opinion on important issues, to appoint one member of the Supervisory Board and to ask the court to discharge a failing supervisor. There is certainly reason to doubt the effectiveness of the voice arrangement. Problems to be considered, for instance, relate to how to ascertain that the newly created stakeholder body will represent the interest of all stakeholders, and whether it can have any effective influence on the organization's strategic and operational governance. The associations of service delivery organizations fear more bureaucracy and policy inertia.

Another important reason to denounce the social enterprise model concerns the position of investors. Investors are given the right to invest in a social enterprise. As a shareholder, they also have a right to be paid a "result-contingent" return on investment. Interestingly, the word "profit" is explicitly avoided, to reflect the non-commercial nature of a social enterprise: profit maximization should never be its purpose. However, external investors should not be in a position to have a determinative influence on the organization's strategic and operational governance. Their only right in this respect is to appoint a representative in the Supervisory Board. The arrangement could not be more hybrid. It reflects the still highly controversial nature of profit-making hospital care in the Netherlands. It is a typical political compromise between contesting views, and is likely to be impracticable in reality.

The new directions discussed in this section indicate that the reinforcement of hospital governance is viewed as an important policy deserving much attention, particularly in a time of significant changes in the regulatory and sociocultural landscape. The eventual outcome of these developments is hard to predict as yet, but it is clear that there are interesting times ahead.

9.6 References

Helderman J-K et al. (2005). Market-oriented health care reforms and policy learning in the Netherlands. *Journal of Health Politics, Policy & Law*, 20(1–2):189–210.

Lodewick L (2008). *Ziekenhuizen veranderen [Changing hospitals]*. Maastricht, MediMan Holding.

Maarse J (1995). Fixed budgets in the inpatient sector: the case of the Netherlands. In: Schwarz F, Glennester H, Saltman R, eds. *Fixing health budgets. Experience from Europe and North America*. Chichester, John Wiley:75–92.

Maarse J, Normand CH (2009). Markets and competition in European hospital care. In: Rechel B et al., eds. *Investing in hospitals of the future*. Copenhagen, WHO Regional Office for Europe on behalf of the European Observatory on Health Systems and Policies:103–123.

Maarse J, Paulus A (2011). The politics of Dutch health care reform after 2006. *Health Economics, Policy and Law*, 6:125–134.

Meurs P, Schraven TH, eds. (2006). *Naar stimulerend and slim toezicht [Towards stimulating and smart supervision]*. Maarssen, Elsevier Gezondheidszorg.

Nederlandse Zorgautoriteit (2009). *Ziekenhuis Monitor 2008 [Hospital monitor]*. Utrecht, Nederlandse Zorgautoriteit.

Tulleneers JP (2010). *Meetlat inkomens bestuurders zorginstellingen 2008 [Measuring income data for executive members of health care provider organizations 2008]*. Maastricht, PC Kwadraat (http://www.bestuurderscentrum.nl/site/publicatie_detail.asp?titel=meetlat_inkomens_bestuurders_zorginstellingen&vid=266, accessed 14 June 2011).

Van de Ven W, Schut F (2008). Universal mandatory health insurance in the Netherlands. *Health Affairs*, 3:371–381.

Chapter 10
Norway

Jon Magnussen

10.1 Introduction: specialized health care in Norway

Norway is a relatively small, sparsely populated country with a population of 4.7 million. It has one of the most expensive health care systems in the world, ranking only behind the United States and Luxembourg in terms of per capita spending (OECD, 2009). Norway belongs to the family of tax-financed health care systems, and has a decentralized governance structure, in keeping with the tradition of a Nordic health care model (Magnussen et al., 2009). A difference between the Norwegian health care system and those of the other Nordic countries, however, is that responsibility for primary and specialized health care services lies at different government levels. Thus, while the 430 municipalities are responsible for primary care, the responsibility for specialized health care is decentralized to four state-owned regional health authorities.

A description and discussion of hospital governance requires a brief introduction to the specific governance structure of the specialized health care system. The present system dates back to 2002 when ownership of hospitals was centralized from 19 counties to the state, and the sector organized into five independent regional health authorities. Thus the reform both represented a re-centralization of ownership and a move from a model of devolution (through elected county councils) to deconcentration (through appointed boards). The reform was motivated through two main goals; a higher level of structural efficiency and the removal of a persistent "blame game" between hospitals, counties and state (for a more thorough discussion see Hagen & Kaarbøe (2006) and Magnussen, Hagen & Kaarbøe (2007)).

The specific content of the reform was to:

- centralize ownership;

- strengthen governance and management through the use of independent health trusts;

- apply the same principles of accounting as those used in private enterprises.

The last point in essence meant that capital costs were included in hospital accounting. The initial model has since been modified in two ways; from 2006 politicians were "reinstated" as board members and in 2007 the number of regional health authorities was reduced from five to four. Notably, however, the reinstatement of politicians does not imply a return to a model of devolution. Regional board members are appointed by the Ministry of Health and Care Services, rather than elected by the public, and local board members are appointed by the regional board.

The state owns the four regional health authorities. Each authority is governed by a Board of Trustees appointed by the Minister of Health and Care Services. The state carries out its strategic and operational governance through the Ministry of Health and Care Services – more specifically, through the Department of Hospital Ownership within the Ministry. This department prepares annual governing documents, recently renamed "task documents", to signal that the central authorities primarily are concerned with strategic rather than operational governance. In addition to the task documents, there is an annual enterprise meeting – similar to the general assembly held in private firms. The Ministry of Health and Care Services describes its governance as "active exercise of ownership … (through) … management requirements related to organizational and financial matters and framework conditions" (Ministry of Health and Care Services, 2010).

One level down, the regional health authorities own the hospitals, and these are organized as *independent* health trusts. Health trusts explicitly are, therefore, independent legal entities with governing bodies (hospital boards) appointed by the regional health authority; these boards have the same mix of politicians and other representatives as the regional boards. There is some variation between the regional health authorities, in terms of who fills the roles as the chairman of the health trusts' boards. While some regional authorities place their own representative as chairman of hospitals boards, other regional health authorities choose an external representative to fill this position. The strategic and operational governance of the health trusts is carried out – as at regional level – through "task documents" and annual enterprise meetings.

There is a clear division of responsibilities and tasks between the state, the regional health authorities and the local health trusts. The regional health authorities are regulated by a set of statutes clearly defining the responsibility of the regional health authorities to "coordinate the activity and division of tasks between the local health trusts in an appropriate and efficient way".[16] The local health trusts also operate under a set of statues regulating (among other things) specific tasks and investment decisions.

While this description may suggest that the regional health authorities are quasi-autonomous bodies, while local health trusts are "independent" only on paper, the picture is in reality somewhat more complex. Some local trusts effectively consist of one hospital, while others represent organizational (and in some cases physical) mergers of several hospitals. In the latter case, local trusts may have substantial autonomy in deciding to redistribute tasks between hospitals. Formally, however, decisions are made at the regional level, and in practice regional health authorities differ in terms of the extent to which they allow local autonomy.

10.2 Strategic governance within the regional health authorities

In the present Norwegian model, the role of the central government is one of strategic governance at national level, as well as laying out the financial and organizational framework within which the sector operates. We now turn to the role of the regional health authorities in the regional strategic governance of the health sector. Three issues are of particular interest: hospital structure, allocation of resources and investment decisions.

As already mentioned, the *structural framework* of hospitals is – in principle – determined by the regional health authority. Thus, the regional health authority makes decisions regarding the broad distribution of clinical services between the independent health trusts in the region. In the case of investment decisions, the same will apply to the location and size of the facilities. In a sparsely populated country such as Norway, however, hospital structure and the distribution of tasks have emerged as a major political issue. The present three-party government coalition, which has been in a majority since 2005, has pledged that "no local hospital shall be shut down". A heated discussion has risen out of this pledge, relating to whether removing acute-care functions from small hospitals in reality implies redefining them as medical centres, as well as whether merging hospitals into larger hospital trusts and then restructuring within the trusts is a way of escaping this pledge. The ambiguity in the interpretation of what

---

16 Author's translation.

exactly constitutes a "local hospital" increases the tension both between the local health trusts and the regional health authority and between the regional health authority and the state. In some cases, the Ministry of Health and Care Services will have views on regional structures and will directly influence the decisions made by the regional boards.

One example provides a good description of the relationship between the board of the regional health authority and the Ministry of Health and Care Services. In the central Norway regional health authority, one of the independent hospital trusts consists of two hospitals located in two cities. One of the hospitals is rather old, the buildings are run down and it is generally acknowledged that there is need for substantial investment. Broadly speaking, there are two options:

1. continue with activity in two locations – that is, build a new hospital while continuing with the existing activity in the hospital in the other city; or

2. close down the existing facilities and build a new, larger hospital that can absorb the activity from both the existing hospitals.

A cost–benefit analysis of the situation gave no clear guidance, partly because the potential for economies of scale is difficult to establish *ex ante* and partly because costs/benefits related to personnel recruitment, travel costs and potential changes in quality are difficult to quantify. After a lengthy, ministry-initiated process in which both the board of the local hospital trust and the board of the regional health authority recommended option 1 (above), the Ministry of Health and Care Services stated that it would not provide investment loans, thus overruling both the local and the regional boards' decision. While the Ministry of Health and Care Services could argue that this stance was based on the ability of the regional health authority to provide its share of the investment costs, the general impression was that the Ministry preferred option 2, but felt that openly saying so would represent direct interference with what should be a regional health authority decision.

Similar examples can be found in other parts of the country. In some cases, local health trusts seem to be able to decide on a division of tasks and a structure within the health trust without the regional health authority or the Ministry of Health and Care Services feeling the need to intervene. In other cases, the regional health authority intervenes, but the Ministry of Health and Care Services does not. A full analysis of which factors trigger regional health authority and/or Ministry of Health and Care Services intervention is beyond the scope of this chapter, but a general message is that there seems to be what could be called a lack of precision in the understanding and use of the terms "strategic" and "operational" governance. Thus, a decision that by some is viewed as "operational" (for example, the merging of maternity wards in two closely located hospitals in order to optimize quality and cost-efficiency), is viewed as "strategic" by others (for example, the issue of whether all acute-care hospitals should include a maternity ward). Furthermore, whether a decision is "strategic" or "operational" obviously depends on its political implications. In the above-mentioned example the subtle ministerial overruling of the regional health authority can be interpreted in the light of the particular political landscape in that local area.

Turning now to the *financial framework* for the hospitals,[17] this is also an area in which decisions are made by the regional health authority. Under the present financing system in Norway, the incomes of regional health authorities are set as a combination of capitation and activity-based financing. The purpose of the capitation model – mostly used within the regional health authorities – is to present financial opportunities for the regional health authorities to provide the same level of services to their populations. Each health trust is associated with a specific catchment area and is allocated its budget as a combination of the estimated relative need of the population of that area and actual activity. These catchment areas are "informal" and in some cases coincide with the "old" county borders, creating a situation of "dual governance" for the hospital management so that they need to focus on both serving the need of a specific population and running the hospital. As few hospitals provide a full set of services, they need to purchase certain services from other hospitals.

A natural question relates to why the regional health authorities prefer to use a capitation-based model rather than a cost–volume type of contract, or a commissioning model. One possible explanation for the use of capitation models within the regional health authorities is that the local health trusts cover geographical areas that are somewhat similar to counties, and using a capitation based model preserves a notion of geographical fairness within the regional health authorities that resembles the old system of financing specialist health care in the counties.

Until the 2002 reform, *funding of investments* and costing of capital were issues resolved independently of the hospital management. Investments were funded by counties or jointly by counties and the central government – in other words, there were no capital costs in the hospital accounting system and the cost of capital for the hospital management was (seemingly) zero. With the hospital reform in 2002, capital costs were included in hospital accounting and the transfer of funds to regional health authorities was expanded to include funds for investments.

---

17 I use the term hospital and independent health trust interchangeably, although the latter may contain more than one hospital.

Initially, there was a substantial discussion regarding the level of funds provided by the state for investments; in 2002 this was set at 60% of depreciation costs, but has since been gradually increased to cover the level of depreciation that followed from the valuation of capital in 2002. Formally, however, the state does not distinguish between funds for investment and funds for operating costs; regional health authorities are, therefore, free to invest, provided they can cover the costs within their budgetary framework. Since regional health authorities can only finance their investments from general funds and loans from the state, however, the level of investments is limited by the availability of loans. Further, these state loans are limited, thus in practice further limiting the investment autonomy of the regional health authorities.

Currently, state loans can be used for large investments up to 50% of total investment costs. The remaining 50% must comprise accumulated surpluses from within the regional health authorities. The interesting implication of this is that an investment (for example, replacing an old building with a new one) that is cost-efficient – in the sense that the increase in capital costs will be offset by a reduction in labour costs – will not be realized unless the regional health authority can provide 50% of the investment costs. In practice, this means that cost-efficient investments will be delayed until regional health authorities can accumulate enough surplus to cover their share. While this may seem puzzling, it reflects the substantial degree of uncertainty attached to cost–benefit analysis of large health care investments, as well as the inherent scepticism at the central level that potential efficiency gains will actually be realized. We note that the central authority only regulates the liquidity – it does not necessarily question the investment decision in itself. However, this is a (perhaps not so) subtle way of limiting the autonomy of the regional health authorities.

There is an ongoing debate regarding how to allocate investment funds *within* the regional health authorities. While some regional health authorities distribute a specific investment budget according to specified board-approved plans, others delegate responsibility for some investment decisions to the health trusts. Thus, decisions relating to smaller investments (for example, in equipment) are more likely to be carried out at local level than larger investments (in buildings, for example). While there is nothing – in theory – to prevent the regional health authorities from decentralizing investment decisions,[18] a centralized investment procedure can be explained in the context of the statutory responsibility of the regional health authorities to coordinate general activity and specific tasks. Local trust autonomy is thereby limited to operating within a capital framework set out by the regional health authority. There are also variations in how funds that are made available as a result of the different timing of actual (re)investment

---

18 Save, of course, the liquidity constraints already discussed.

and allocation of resources are handled.[19] If funds that are made available from one health trust are used to finance investments in another trust, some regional health authorities impose an interest rate on these funds, while others do not.

10.3 Operational governance: general features and a specific case

I now turn to the question of operational governance, focusing on the hospital (health trust) level and using a specific health trust as an illustrative example.

The trust chosen, St Olavs Hospital Trust, is one of five (regional) teaching hospitals in Norway. It is located in the central Norway regional health authority, where it serves partly as a local hospital for the town of Trondheim (with a population of 160 000), partly as a central hospital for the Sør-Trøndelag county (270 000 people) and partly as a highly specialized regional hospital for the three counties Møre og Romsdal, Sør Trøndelag and Nord Trøndelag (with a combined population of 550 000, some 12% of the total population of Norway). St Olavs Hospital Trust has an operating budget in excess of Norwegian krone (NKr) 6500 million, with a staff comprising about 4700 person years.

During the period 1999–2011, St Olavs Hospital was completely rebuilt, with old buildings torn down and replaced by new and modern facilities and others completely renovated, representing a total investment of about NKr 12.5 billion,[20] or the equivalent of two years' operating expenses at 2008 prices. Financing has come in part from special grants from the government and in part from the regional health authorities' own investment funds and general income.

There has been a substantial amount of tension between the hospital, the regional health authority and the central government over who should be responsible for the funding of the project. Since St Olavs Hospital consumes around half of the total budget for the central Norway regional health authority, the substantial investment in this hospital has also created a lot of tension within the region. Fig. 10.1 shows St Olavs Hospital deficits for the period 2004–2009.

By the end of 2005, the hospital was clearly out of control, financially. The Minister of Health and Care Services (representing the Labour Party) publicly stated that the board and management did not take the economic situation with sufficient seriousness. In the spring of 2006, both the CEO and the chairman of the board resigned, and by the end of the year the CEO of the regional health

---

19 An example of this can be observed in the difference between capital costs and capital expenses. When the former exceeds the latter, this generates liquidity that can be used within the regional health authority.

20 €1 = NKr 7.8 (average for 2010 – see Oanda currency conversion web site (http://www.oanda.com/currency/historical-rates/, accessed 14 June 2011)).

Fig. 10.1 *St Olavs Hospital deficits, 2004–2009*

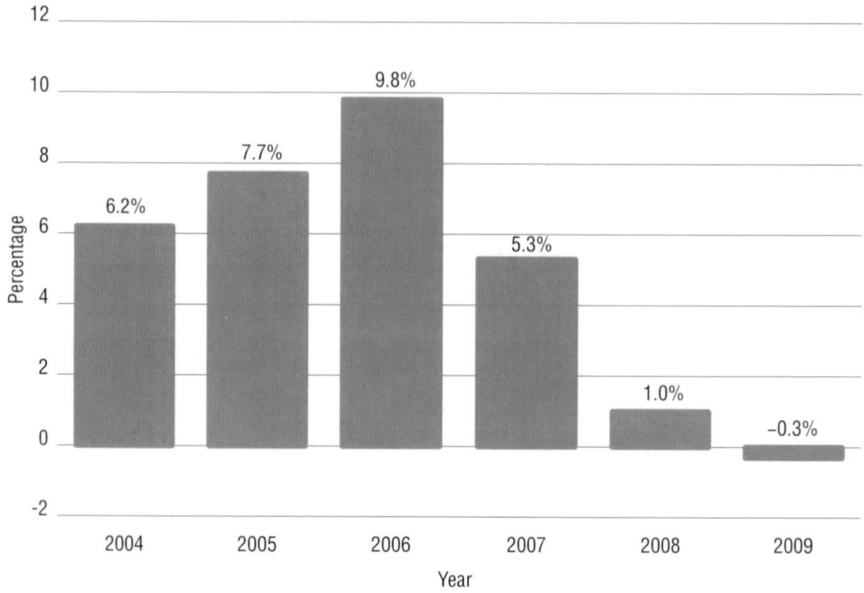

authority also asked to be relieved of his duties. Although the resignations were not officially related to the deficit, it is fair to assume that the pressure created by the economic situation played some role. At the end of 2006, the deficit had reached a staggering 10% of total hospital costs. In the three-year period that followed, however, this deficit was first halved and then eliminated.

Attributing the change in economic performance solely to the change in management would be an unjust simplification. External factors – such as the growth in aggregate health care spending and the gradual transition from running a hospital in two parallel environments ("old and new") to operating in new and functional buildings – are likely to have played important roles. The economic performance of the hospital, however, provides a useful background for our description of specific operational governance issues. Looking at how operational governance is practised in a health trust under extreme economic pressure also illustrates to what extent the ambitions of the reform as a "management and leadership reform" (Magnussen, Hagen & Kaarbøe, 2007) have been fulfilled.

The following sections briefly consider some key questions of operational governance. While St Olavs Hospital is the most frequently used example, we occasionally refer to how different regional health authorities approach governance issues in different ways. The first relevant question is whether there are established *limits or boundaries that restrict hospital and/or management decisions* which do not follow formally defined corporate goals and objectives set at the political level. Put another way: to what extent to management have to "play it by ear" relative to often vaguely formulated political goals?

To understand to what extent there might be implicit or explicit boundaries, it is illustrative to briefly consider the corporate goals as described in the task (governing) document from the regional health authority. For St Olavs Hospital, this document describes the budget allocation, including the amount of resources available for the hospital, and the expected financial result ("balanced budget"). It also describes overall goals related to activity and quality. Some of the parameters used in governance are described in Table 10.1.

Table 10.1 *Governance variables*

Governance variables
Number of casemix-adjusted discharges
Income from outpatient activity (proxy for outpatient activity)
Share of patients in mental health care admitted against their own will
Share of cases sent to the "Norwegian system for compensation to patients", in which patients have been favoured
Share of waiting times published on the Internet that have been updated in the past two weeks
At least 80% of patient medical records sent to GPs within two weeks after discharge
No patients staying in the corridor
Patients should have an individual plan
Share of acute-care readmissions with two weeks in mental health care
Share of caesarean sections
Less than 5% of planned surgeries should be cancelled
Number of consultations per day in psychiatric care should increase
Average waiting time should not increase for somatic care and should be reduced for psychiatric care and substance abuse-related care
Waiting time for assessment for mental health care under the age of 18 years should be less than 10 days

As noted in section 10.1, the regional health authority will receive a similar document from its owner, the Ministry of Health and Care Services, and several of the goals presented therein will simply be passed on to the hospital. An important difference, however, is that while the regional health authority receives a "task" document, the health trust receives a "governing" document, implying that the governance at this level is more detailed than at regional level.

The task document describes goals related to a number of broadly defined patient-related activities. Yet, it is fair to say that the most important goals relating to the practical governance of the regional health authority include the level of activity and the financial result. Thus, within the explicit boundaries set by the budget and the (more implicit) distribution of functions to hospitals, we would assume that regional governance imposes few limits or boundaries on the management of the hospital.

There are, however, several examples of such boundaries – most related to a (re) structuring of the hospital – aiming to reduce operational costs and achieve budget balance. They also illustrate that, contrary to how it is supposed to behave, the Ministry of Health and Care Services actively engages in the operational governance of the sector.

10.3.1 Example 1: IVF

In two public reports (NOU 1987, 1997) central authorities in Norway attempted to provide criteria for prioritizing among patient groups. In both cases, IVF was an example of a type of health care service considered to fall outside the boundaries of the public health care sector responsibility. When St Olavs Hospital looked closely in 2006 at the possibility of reducing the level of some services to obtain budget balance, IVF was, therefore, a natural choice. The amount of money saved was comparatively small, but the significance of reducing the level of services for a low-priority group of patients was considerable.

The regional health authority, however, did not accept this solution. Furthermore, the "No" from the regional health authority came as a direct result of a "No" from the Minister of Health and Care Services. The political pressure of having to deal with the patient interest groups (who – of course – received a great deal of support from opposition politicians) was simply too high. The plan was abandoned by the hospital management within a few days of first being proposed.

10.3.2 Example 2: elective orthopaedic surgery in a remote local hospital

St Olavs Hospital operates out of three different locations; most of the activity is carried out in Trondheim (population of around 160 000), some local hospital functions are performed 35 minutes away in Orkdal (with a population of 11 000) and elective orthopaedic surgery is performed in Røros (with a population of 5500), more than two hours' driving distance from Trondheim. Furthermore, since the majority of patients treated in Røros come from the Trondheim area, maintaining activity in Røros implies moving patients and physicians from Trondheim to Røros and back again. Conservative estimates made in 2006/2007 suggested that closing down Røros could lead to a potential saving of around NKr 25 million.

Why, then, was health care activity still being carried out in Røros when St Olavs Hospital had to remove a deficit of almost NKr 600 million? The obvious answer lies in the characterization of the hospital as a "local hospital". As mentioned earlier, in the parliamentary period 2005–2009 the government stated explicitly that no local hospital would be shut down. Since Røros is not a hospital entity, but rather a part of the larger independent trust of St Olavs Hospital, this should not affect any management decision to close down the facility. Knowing, however, that any attempt to close down the facility would be blocked by the Ministry of Health and Care Services (formally by the board of the regional health authority), the facility was allowed to remain open, and the saving of NKr 25 million was realized in other areas.[21]

Two discussion points arise from these examples.

1. First, overruling the hospital management on the IVF issue did not substantially increase the challenge of achieving a balance between income and costs, since the potential cost savings were relatively minor. It meant, however, that the autonomy and legitimacy of the management was seriously questioned; within the organization, the message received was that "the management tried, but was overruled". There is a possibility that this may reduce the likelihood of further cost-reducing proposals being implemented. In particular, it may imply that cutting budgets across the board is a more a feasible strategy for management than selecting areas with low priority and/or low cost-efficiency.

2. Second, while "lost savings" due to these (more or less) subtle interventions by the state are not essential to obtain a balanced budget, the intervention still represents a distraction for the management, pulling its attention away from operational management and towards a search for solutions that might appease the politicians involved.

An additional area of analysis is the extent to which the hospital management team is allowed to *organize its own internal operational structures* (architecture and routines – operational methodology, clearly mapped processes, benchmarks/best practice standards, etc.), something that also relates to who defines authority and responsibility, as well as whether the management of the hospital can make decisions affecting professional structures (e.g. numbers and functions of chiefs of service).

---

21 It should be noted that these were not strategic decisions, in the sense that they came as a result of "who would do what, where and why", but rather as a result of the need to balance the budget – thus, the question for hospital management was "how can we adjust the way we operate the hospital so that we can balance the budget?" Notably, the climate has lately changed in favour of shifting the activity focus of the hospital to less-specialized services, effectively turning it into a health centre.

St Olavs Hospital has complete freedom in this regard, within the boundaries laid out in the governing document and under the assumption that the hospital board will sanction the chosen model. It is also worth noting that this issue seems to be uncontroversial, which is not surprising if we bear in mind that the hospital reform in 2002 was marketed as a "responsibility and leadership reform" (before 2002 this was an area in which hospitals were required to adapt to a set of centrally imposed restrictions, clearly limiting the flexibility of the management).

The fact that the issue is uncontroversial does not mean, however, that the results are uncontroversial within the organization. Attempts by the central management in St Olavs Hospital to restructure the clinical departments have not been successful due to internal "opposition". Other independent health trusts have also faced serious internal opposition when attempting to restructure the distribution of services and "redraw" the organizational map of the hospital, something that could (should?), however, be viewed as an example of a decentralized governance model that is actually working.

By comparison the concept of "departmentalization" becomes more controversial when departments are created across physical structures, or even across different geographical locations. As already described, one consequence of the 2002 hospital reform has been that the local health trusts now sometimes encompasses several hospitals located in different cities. In some cases these have a history of (more or less) friendly rivalry (Magnussen, 1994), and the merger into one organization has not always been easy. There might also be substantial geographical differences that limit the choices available to the hospital management. This is accentuated by the composition of the local boards, in that local politicians will often look out for the interests of their own constituency rather than the interest of the health trust as a whole. In interviews with managers in local health trusts comprising several hospitals in different geographical locations, a picture emerges in which they are autonomous as long as they stay within budget and do not propose changes that provoke opposition from local or central politicians. The core dilemma here relates to which decisions could (should?) be administratively decentralized and which should be politically (de)centralized.

St Olavs Hospital practises what could be termed a decentralized model of internal governance in terms of the extent to which the *responsibility for objectives corresponds with decision capacity*. There are approximately 300 individuals on "level 2 and level 3", who make hiring decisions and are allowed to purchase "non-expensive" equipment. A specific budget is allocated for medium-sized equipment at level 2 (clinics), while the larger investment decisions are made centrally. The difference between the degree of decentralization relating to hiring versus investment decisions must be understood in terms of the long-term consequences of each; while investments are largely "sunk costs", the use of personnel is closely monitored and thus higher-level management can intervene in the case of deviations between actual and budgeted levels of employment. Also, it should be noted, hiring decisions may be temporarily centralized when there are more severe economic difficulties. The setting up of new clinical trials, however, needs to be discussed within the combined group of clinical chiefs.

The case of Oslo University Hospital – by far the largest hospital in Norway, with over 22 000 employees and a total budget of NKr 18 billion – provides another illustration worth mentioning. The hospital is the result of a merger of three teaching hospitals in the Oslo area. There are persistent problems with deficits, and in the autumn of 2009 the management chose to centralize to the level of the CEO all hiring decisions, all investment decisions and all decisions regarding using consultants. In the long term this is clearly an inefficient method of hospital governance, but it reflects the challenges faced by hospital management when the organization is not culturally equipped to handle budget responsibility.

Regarding *monitoring and follow up*, Norwegian hospitals have full autonomy in deciding on the parameters for monitoring day-to-day activity, provided they report to the regional health authority on the parameters specified in the governing document. Information is provided on a hierarchical basis; that is, the type of information will depend on the position within the organization of the party that receiving the information. Most information is available on a monthly basis, although the organization expresses a preference for more frequent updates, preferably on a weekly basis. What is reported and what is regarded as important information will vary within as well as between hospitals, but these issues do not tend to be the subject of much conflict.

An interesting question in terms of hospital governance in Norway is that no *incentive schemes* have been implemented. Employees are on fixed salaries, with extra payments for long hours or extra shifts, and there are no performance-related incentive schemes. Salary levels are primarily set in central negotiations, and although there is some space for local discretion, most professions follow "national norms" (a more individual approach to wage setting would not be accepted by unions). After the 2002 reform, the responsibility for wage negotiations was transferred to the Employers Association for enterprises with public association, but attempts to generate a more individual model for setting wage levels have not been successful. Performance indicators are there for management (at all levels) but not for the employees, and they are not differentiated in organizational or group terms.

10.4 Conclusions: some key dilemmas

The discussion in the previous sections highlights some of the key features of the Norwegian model of hospital governance; a three-level model with a high degree of decentralization but within some (often not explicitly stated) political boundaries. Within this structure there are, however, some key dilemmas.

First we note that there is a dilemma between a model based on centralized ownership and decentralized management justified by a perception of "better and more professional management". Thus, the Norwegian model is formally "quasi-autonomous" in the sense that regional health authorities are given a great deal of autonomy and the state is meant to govern primarily through the financial and structural framework. Yet, there seems to be a perception both by regional and local health authorities that the degree of central regulation in some cases overrides the possibility to make astute local decisions.

This dilemma also translates to the relationship between the regional health authorities and the local hospital trusts. While the statutes of the regional health authorities clearly state that they are responsible for making decisions that obviously affect the local health trusts (division of tasks, details relating to the financing system, large investment decisions), the intention of the model is to leave the local hospital trusts with some autonomy to run their operations within the framework provided by the regional health authority. In this case, it seems fair to say that local health trusts are autonomous when it comes to internal institutional arrangements, internal financial matters and, to some extent, accountability arrangements.

This conclusion, however, requires an interpretation of "autonomous" as "within a centrally set broad structural and financial framework". Thus, local health trusts are not free to introduce new services or to discard old ones, but they are (mostly) free to organize the delivery of those services for which they are made responsible by the regional health authority. In addition, while they cannot determine the mechanism that generates income, or the size of the budget, they are free to organize their internal flow of funds, and internal resource allocation mechanisms. In this sense, the hospital reform in 2002 can be seen as an improvement, as the detailed day-to-day governing of hospitals has been replaced by a governance structure whereby the focus is on results rather than use of inputs.

The current Norwegian model is in its tenth year (2011) and is supported by the present government, but there is an open question regarding whether it will survive the next general election in 2013. All political parties currently in opposition, as well as two out of three coalition partners in the current government, have stated that they see clear weaknesses in the model and would like to see it replaced. A more centralized model in which the regional health authorities are abolished would be most likely to replace it. Local health trusts would then answer directly to the central government. In this case, structural issues – including those relating to investment levels – would be more centralized than they are today. That said, it is difficult to see how a centralized administration ("national directorate of health") would be able to govern local health trusts comprehensively, and so one might expect the level of local autonomy to rise.

10.5 References

Hagen TP, Kaarbøe O (2006). The Norwegian hospital reform of 2002: central government takes over ownership of public hospitals. *Health Policy*, (76):320–333.

Magnussen J (1994). Hospital efficiency in Norway: a nonparametric analysis. *Dissertations in Economics*, 6.

Magnussen J, Hagen TP, Kaarbøe O (2007). Centralized or decentralized? A case study of Norwegian hospital reform. *Social Science and Medicine*, 64(10):2129–2137.

Magnussen J et al. (2009). The Nordic model of health care. In: Magnussen J, Vrangbæk K, Saltman R, eds. *Nordic health care systems: recent reforms and current policy challenges*. Maidenhead, Open University Press:3–30.

Ministry of Health and Care Services (2010). The department of hospital ownership [web site]. Oslo, Ministry of Health and Care Services (http://www.regjeringen.no/en/dep/hod/About-the-Ministry/org/Departments/the-department-of-hospital-ownership.html?id=1413, accessed 22 June 2011).

NOU (1987). *Retningslinjer for prioriteringe innen Norsk helsetjeneste [Guidelines for priority setting in Norwegian health care]*. Oslo, Norwegian Ministry of Health and Care Services (Official Norwegian Reports 25).

NOU (1997). *Prioriteringer på ny [Priority setting again]*. Oslo, Norwegian Ministry of Health and Care Services (Official Norwegian Reports 17).

OECD (2009). Health Data 2009 [online database]. Paris, Organisation for Economic Co-operation and Development (http://www.oecd.org/document/54/0,3343,en_2649_37407_43220022_1_1_1_1,00.html, accessed March 2010).

Chapter 11
Portugal

Vítor M. dos Reis Raposo and Ana P. de Jesus Harfouche

11.1 Introduction

11.1.1 The Portuguese health care system and main hospital reforms

In reality the Portuguese health system includes three coexisting, overlapping subsystems:

1. the NHS;

2. special public and private insurance schemes for certain professions, compulsory for groups of employees; and

3. private voluntary health insurance.

Public sector funding as a share of total expenditure on health care fluctuates around 72%. The NHS, created in 1979 and primarily funded through taxation, is defined in the Portuguese Constitution as "universal, comprehensive and approximately free of charge". It establishes "the right of all citizens to health protection; a guaranteed universal right to health care (mostly free at the point of use) and access for all citizens regardless of economic and social background".

Since the year 2000, hospital care has been subject to two types of reforms: corporatization of public hospitals, with changes made to the public hospital management rules and payment systems; and a redefinition of the existing NHS supply of hospital services, resulting in the closing of several hospital maternity departments, allegedly on clinical safety grounds; putting two or more nearby hospitals under the same management team to reorganize hospital care within the regions; and announcing the building of new hospitals under public–private partnership schemes.

More than a right or wrong, left or right ideology-driven health system reform, policy and political choices have been a vivid expression of the values of contemporary Portuguese society regarding individual and collective rights. Historical facts can be cited to explain the current form and structures as signs of societal respect and appreciation for a number of doctrinal principles. In fact, corporatization is seen as a driver for efficiency and has received great emphasis in recent years, supplemented more recently by some emphasis on quality improvement.

Currently, four types of hospitals coexist in Portugal:

*   PEEHs (*Hospitais EPE*) – these are public institutions, endowed with corporate entity, as well as administrative, financial and patrimonial autonomy and an enterprise nature;

*   administrative public sector hospitals (APSHs) (*Hospitais SPA*) – these are public institutions, endowed with legal personality, as well as administrative and financial autonomy, with or without patrimonial autonomy (traditional public hospitals with public administration); and

*   public–private partnership hospitals (PPPHs) – these are PFIs with the award of two contracts (infrastructure construction and maintenance, and clinical activities management, respectively); and

*   private hospitals.

By 2010, there were 42 PEEHs, 20 APSHs and 3 PPPHs in operation in Portugal. Since the PPPHs are rather few and new,[22] – with not enough long-term activity for thorough assessment as yet – they will not be studied in detail in this chapter; we only mention the main feautures of PPPHs and mostly focus on PEEH hospitals.

11.2 PPPHs

The first attempt to set up a PPPH project in Portugal took place in 2003, inspired by PFIs in the United Kingdom some years earlier. For procedural reasons, however, the goal to build a new hospital on the outskirts of Lisbon failed to move to the final stage of negotiations and subsequent contract signing; recognizing that procedures and proposals were not standardized enough to allow a clear decision to be made, the process had to be restarted. Meanwhile, other private patient partnership projects have been launched and are under review.

---

22 Despite the fact that the process was initiated in 2003, building the first hospital only began in 2008.

An important distinction in the Portuguese PPPHs is the awarding of one contract for infrastructure construction and maintenance, and another for clinical activities management. The current government is still defining a specific format for contracting clinical activities management in a second wave of (six) hospitals (from an initial round of ten new hospitals to be built under the PPPH system). This experience is characterized by a lengthy administrative process of creation derived from the rather complex model adopted, coupled with technical unpreparedness of the public sector on the one hand and an overly ideological discussion, often resulting in distorted views regarding what should/should not be expected from this solution in the health sector, on the other. The partnerships represent a continuous process of advancing and retreating that recently earned harsh criticism from the Court of Auditors regarding delays, the model chosen and the lack of control by the state (Court of Auditors, 2009).

11.2.1 Corporatization of public hospitals

The corporatization of public hospitals was carried out in two waves. The first started in 2002 with the publication of legislation on a new legal hospital management system.[23] By 1 January 2003, about half of the hospitals had been transformed into public companies, with capital provided solely by the Government (hence the name *Hospitais SA*). The approach has been extended to other hospitals over the years. Those that did not go through this transformation process (APSHs) continue to be run according to civil service rules.

Increasing costs in the hospital sector (greater than the growth of services rendered to the population) is one of the key issues behind the need for structural reform. For example, from 1999 to 2001, the budgets of the 40 largest Portuguese hospitals increased by about 26.5%, but "service production" in many of them increased only slightly and in some cases stalled. The increase in total NHS costs from 1995 to 2001 (six years) by around €3 billion, without a proportional improvement in the quality of the health care provided to the population, is also noted as being a major problem, together with a perception that some health professionals had a poor attitude regarding the careful and rigorous use of funds allocated to the NHS. The need not to endanger quality and timely delivery of care to the population and the lack of competitive mechanisms and benchmarking between units, were also taken into account.

By early 2002, the health system seemed to be immobilized and without goals, with scarce efficiency in resource use across the board presenting problems. Structural reform was initiated in April 2002, with fundamental objectives

---

23 Law No. 27/2002.

including quality of care, improvement of access and freedom of choice, efficiency maximization and total spending control.

The structural reform had the following main objectives:

- introducing a "new culture" of business management (based on the philosophy of NPM), promoting policies of monitoring and accountability for results;

- facilitating, with more autonomy and flexibility, unit management at various levels, namely in financing, human resources, supply, operational management and investment management (capital);

- public deficit containment and efficiency promotion;

- introducing a new funding model based on actual hospital "production" (delivery of health care services);

- increasing focus on quality provision and user-centred management policies.

The specific measures adopted included those listed here.

- Corporatization of public *Hospitais SA* to be managed like businesses and given greater autonomy and flexibility, as well as greater decision-making capacity through decentralization of responsibilities and a new legal framework. The strategy was to set up initially a significant number (roughly half) of corporate public hospitals as a "critical mass" that would "infect" the entire sector with their way of working.

- Improving performance in other non-corporate public hospitals (APSHs) through the adoption of best management practices tested in *Hospitais SA*.

- Introducing some benchmarking between *Hospitais SA* and APSHs.

During the first wave of corporatization the political and civil discussion revolved around the reasons for chosing this model and the dangers of privatization. For the second wave of corporatization, since the 2005 elections, the new government[24] wanted to make it clear that hospital privatization was not on the political agenda and changed the name to PEEHs[25] or *Hospitais EPE*, although the management rules had undergone virtually no change relative to the former *Hospitais SA*.

---

24 The first wave of corporatization (2002–2005) occurred under a Social Democratic Government and the second one (since 2005) under a Socialist Government. Those parties have different views in relation to the NHS and the roles of the state and the private sector in health care (more liberal, pro-privatization in the former than in the latter). The specific format of the PEEHs seems to have removed the existing fear of public hospital privatization that was present during 2002–2005 (in fact, such fear was one of the reasons mentioned for adopting the chosen statute, best suited to providing public service).

25 Decree-law No. 233/2005.

The objectives included the expansion of PEEH status to more hospitals, as well as creating hospital centres[26] (concentration) and local health unities[27] (integration of care). Emphasis was placed on providing autonomy and management accountability to hospital boards as part of a general trend towards an effective purchaser–provider split. Later in 2007, explicit service contracting was introduced for both PEEHs and APSHs.

11.3 PEEHs

As already indicated, this chapter pays most attention to the PEEHs. The focus is on the institutional, financial and accountability arrangements sustaining their innovative, autonomous approaches, as well as the degree to which the hospital is allowed to honour its autonomy in practice in operational terms.

11.3.1 Institutional arrangements

Defined by law as public institutions endowed with corporate identity, administrative, financial and patrimonial autonomy and an enterprise nature,[28] different criteria are used in the process of transforming a traditional APSH into a PEEH. The corporatization process is initiated by a voluntary decision on the part of hospital and the main criteria used are size, type of activity and regional representation.

Ownership is public and the legal framework is defined by government regulation, through a specific statute[29] generic to all hospitals, which must follow the strategic orientation and goals defined for the NHS. The location and size of the PEEH are set centrally by the main shareholder, the state, represented by the Ministry of Finance and the Ministry of Health. The two ministries have strategic trusteeship and oversight of each PEEH. As the main shareholders, their principal functions are as follows.

- Approve work plans and budgets. The Regional Health Administration (RHA) and the Central Health System Administration (CAHS) (previously called the Institute for Financial Management and Informatics) start the process by asking every hospital to submit their proposals for the following year, usually carried out by August/September. The RHA and the CAHS analyse the proposals, considered within the total budget given by the Ministers of Finance and Health, and negotiate with each hospital the

---

26 A group of reorganized hospitals in a region in which each hospital has no administrative and financial autonomy, shares the management team and has common services and functional links.

27 Formed by a hospital and a group of primary care health centres, its main objective is to integrate both levels of care. They have the same management team, some common services and functional links.

28 According to Decree-law No. 558/99 and article no. 18 from the annex of Law No. 27/2002.

29 Decree-law No. 233/2005.

final terms of their budgets. After negotiation, they submit the budget for the Ministries' approval.

- Approve the accounting documents. Each hospital sends its annual report for approval by the Ministry of Health and the Ministry of Finance, which is usually given after the Directorate-General of Treasury and Finance (DGTF) analyses and approves the document.

- Authorize the purchases and sales of buildings, as well as their encumbrance. This is carried out by the DGTF verifying the financial and operational aspects of the transaction.

- Authorize, according to the advice and approval of the auditor, the execution of investments when the global matching funds are not provided within the approved budgets and the amount exceeds 2% of registered capital. The process begins with the hospital sending an authorization request to the DGTF, accompanied by the expressed opinion of the auditor. The DGTF then issues an opinion and sends it for the ministries' approval, usually granted if the cost–benefit of the investment is well documented.

- Determine the increases and reductions in hospital registered capital.

- Authorize the raising of loans, the individual or total value of which are equal to or greater than 10% of registered capital. A public fund has recently been created to reduce interest rates to be paid by hospitals in case they need to raise loans.

- Authorize transfers of hospital services in partnership with other public entities for the better carrying out of the PEEH objectives.

- Authorize the participation of hospitals in other limited companies ("anonymous societies", with capital mostly owned by the hospital) in the field of health care provision.

- Authorize other actions requiring ministry approval as per the applicable law, such as seting up hospital user fees or updating the table price related to DRG health services, and so on.

Internal organizational rules and regulations – as well as non-statutory aspects, including the creation of appropriate governing bodies adjusted to their specificity, size and complexity – are left for the hospital Administration Board (AB) to define. Each PEEH has an AB comprising a president and a maximum of up to six (usually four) members, depending on size and complexity of the hospital. AB members are appointed by joint order of the Ministry of Finance and the Ministry of Health from among individuals of recognized merit and appropriate profile. As a legal requirement, two of those members must be a clinical director and a nurse director, the former a physician and the latter a nurse. If one of the members or the president is a medical doctor by profession, s/he can also assume the post of clinical director, as has been the case in some smaller hospitals in particular. A non-executive member may also be appointed by the same procedure if proposed by the municipality in which the head PEEH office is located.

The AB is appointed for renewable periods of three years. In practice, while some AB members remain in office for successively renewed mandates, other ABs have experienced constant upheaval on the board for political or other reasons. A previous study of four APSHs and four types of PEEH (Raposo, 2007) found a high AB rotation between 2000 and 2007, with 22 different ABs across all hospitals, 32 different presidents and 37 different executive members; just two hospitals had the same board since the year 2000; four had seen three different ABs and two others had seen four ABs. As a rule, the AB meets weekly, whenever called upon by the president and at the request of either two of its members or the auditor. Decisions are made by simple majority vote, with the president holding a quality vote. Minutes containing the summary of proceedings and any voting that takes place must be recorded, the contents must be transcribed and corrected, and the final document signed during the next meeting.

In principle, the PEEH statute gives the AB autonomy to define clinical service levels, provided they do not affect free access to services by the patients. General public hospitals (including PEEHs) are supposed to serve their geographical areas as part of a network in which patients are referred to alternative hospitals according to specialties. Supported by an interinstitutional integrated information system, this *hospital referral network* provides the means for mutual complementarity and technical support relationships, with the objective to ensure patient access to health care providers. The Hospital Referral Networks are, in practice, a set of medical specialties and technologies resulting from a population health needs approach to strategic planning by the Ministry of Health on the basis of distribution ratios and predefined facilities, equipment and human resources. In other words, hospitals are allowed to set up specialties, develop expertise and serve the population within a range of services offered, but they cannot create any new services departing from the logic associated with Hospital Referral Network without permission from the Ministry of Health. Considering both the traditional obedience of politically appointed ABs and the existence of Hospital Referral Networks, it could be concluded that, in practice, ABs have little autonomy to define new services.

Internal organization has, in general, a "cascade management" logic, led by the AB, which, in principle, is entitled to make decisions affecting professional structures (for example, regarding numbers and functions of service directors). It could also decide, for example, to decentralize powers, giving services greater autonomy and responsibility. The scope for participation and intervention by heads of clinical services depends on the delegation of AB powers and is very variable (including the possibility to delegate powers to non-members under their supervision). The AB may also decide on the degree of decision-making autonomy – that is, whether decisions can be made by any particular member or should only be adopted at an AB meeting. The management of the hospital (AB plus CEO) has freedom to arrange clinical trials, which is vital for training and research hospitals. This is often carried out in collaboration with external actors, such as pharmaceuticals companies or the European Organization for Research and Treatment of Cancer.

Hospitals have a number of functional units, aggregations of specialized human resources and technology, integrated services or departments acting as technical support committees to advise the AB on selected matters, on its own initiative or upon request. Some are compulsory (e.g. the aforementioned ethical matters, humane treatment and service quality, nosocomial infection control, pharmacy and therapeutics, certification of termination of pregnancy), while others may be created by the AB (e.g. monitoring and recovery of waiting times; safety, hygiene and health at work; interdepartmental monitoring and evaluation), reflecting their structure, composition and operation in the internal regulations of the hospital. The technical support committees are also important as part of the internal control system and in ensuring proper risk management as an ongoing, interactive and fluid activity throughout the organization. The AB also possesses the autonomy to define through internal regulation (following a proposal of the clinical director) the composition of clinical committees and to appoint their chairmen.

The statutes of all public hospitals (corporatized or traditional) attach great importance to the involvement of medical staff. A previous study (Raposo, 2007) including questions related to the topic found that the physicians' participation is high in terms of surgery block management but limited in decisions regarding recruitment of additional staff and in the area of planning responses to the health needs of the population. Such participation was measured in terms of the integration of doctors in the AB, relations with department managers and heads of service, participation in intermediate management levels or involvement with technical support committees.

The involvement of private actors is also subject to specific statutory rules. A PEEH may establish, for example, an individual services contract with any private physician to perform a given type of surgery with the aim of maximizing the use of the surgery block, but prior permission of the Ministry of Health would be needed for a private entrepreneur to create a specific clinic service within the hospital. Indoor pharmacies in public hospitals are the only case allowed to date, subject to specific legal requirements.[30] The AB has autonomy to hire private ambulance services to transport patients between different centres, as well as to create dedicated services to move professionals, products and materials between different centres by their own means or using private transport services. This same service can be used to transport users whose health status would not require an ambulance, and the same applies to renting space for other types of service, for example, bars, restaurants, financial institutions, vending machines or parking areas, among others – already common practice among the PEEHs. Similar arrangements can be made for various support resources, such as cleaning services.

Workers in corporatized PEEHs are subject to employment contracts, according to the Labour Code, other labour laws, mandatory rules regarding professional titles, collective regulation of working arrangements and internal regulations. The PEEH staff statute provides transition solutions between the traditional public employment, civil servant contract of the past and a regular labour contract (transitional scheme, scheme of permanent option, option scheme and temporary mobility scheme/service commission). In the other cases, the AB has the freedom to decide the status of the new staff. Generally speaking, NHS professionals are permitted to carry out private activity (unless it would "result in charges for the NHS to provide care to beneficiaries") and to decide whether or not to be unionized (and if so, which union(s) to join).[31]

According to the legislation on AB responsibilities, a systematic failure in the objectives of quality and efficiency may eventually lead to their dismissal. In theory, therefore, ABs could be dismissed in the case of severe non-compliance; however, there are no known cases of this. A possible explanation beyond the political nature of their appointment (the most immediate explanation for this fact) may be that the contracts are a recent practice (since 2007) and a learning process for both contracting partners while tools to support and monitor the process are developed. It is assumed that over the coming years the limits of the formal rules will be more firmly implemented, and the system will become more rigid.

AB members themselves feel that they lack autonomy – especially in strategic planning – in some financial areas, including in capital (investment), in terms of the definition of performance targets and to a greater extent regarding supplies and human resources. Their impression is that they spend too much time with bureaucratic issues considered "not very important" or "somewhat important",

---

30 Decree-Law No. 235/2006.

31 Professions may have more than one union.

and very little or little time in strategic planning and quality management, rightly considered "very" or "extremely important" (Raposo, 2007).

11.3.2 Financial arrangements

The financial framework of PEEHs is defined in their statute, under the custody of both the Ministry of Finance and the Ministry of Health. The statutory registered capital is held by the state and may be increased or reduced by joint order of both Ministries. In terms of investment capital, as explained, the hospital is allowed to raise loans to finance investments according to the decision of the AB, up to the limits of 2% and 10% of the registered capital. Outside those limits, the process requires in addition the expression of a favourable opinion from the auditor, and the Ministry of Finance and Ministry of Health as custody shareholders then decide. Operational capital includes revenue from the NHS, mainly raised through the aforementioned programme contract and other "own" revenues from private insurance companies and health subsystems.

Public APSHs and PEEHs sign annually a state budget-funded contract[32] (on average, about 80% of annual hospital revenues) framed by the National Framework Contract Programme (programme contract). The programme contract covers a period of three years, subject to annual reviews, and is followed on a regular basis by the relevant RHA. Hospital budgets were traditionally based on the previous year's funding, updated to allow for inflation; since 1997, a growing fraction has been based on DRGs and on non-adjusted hospital outpatient volumes. The methodology for such programme contracts is published each year as guidelines allocating global budgets through the CAHS,[33] in most cases as a top-down process (from CAHS to AB) with only a limited amount of residual bottom-up capacity for the AB to influence the final result.

By signing the programme contract the hospital commits to certain levels of production by activity/production line, including hospital discharges, outpatient consultations, day-care sessions, ambulatory and inpatient surgical procedures and emergency episodes. Other lines of activity particular to certain hospitals include oncology or psychiatry, prenatal diagnosis, continued care, and prosthetics, among others. Payment is based on work carried out according

---

32 In accordance with the XXXIII base of the Law No. 48/90 (Health Act) with changes introduced by Decree-law No. 27/2002 (new legal regime of hospital management).

33 The CAHS web site provdes useful information (http://www.acss.min-saude.pt, accessed 18 June 2011), in particular:
• information relating to health list prices (http://www.acss.min-saude.pt/DownloadsePublica%C3%A7%C3%B5es/ TabelaseImpressos/Pre%C3%A7osdoSNS/tabid/141/language/pt-PT/Default.aspx, accessed 18 June 2011);
• information on user fees (http://www.acss.min-saude.pt/DownloadsePublica%C3%A7%C3%B5es/TabelaseImpressos/ TaxasModeradoras/tabid/142/language/pt-PT/Default.aspx, accessed 18 June 2011);
• information relating to PEEH contract programmes – guidelines, methodology and final contracts (http://www.acss. min-saude.pt/DownloadsePublica%C3%A7%C3%B5es/HospitaisEPEeSPA/HospitaisEPE/tabid/129/language/pt-PT/ Default.aspx, accessed 18 June 2011).

to baseline prices for each group of hospitals, rather than reimbursing costs incurred. Prices are set by the buyer, requiring the provider unit to achieve predetermined efficiency levels without compromising quality (Ferreira et al., 2010).

The programme contract establishes performance objectives with targets relating to specific indicators at national (quality, access, production, economic and financial performance) and regional (economic and financial performance and other regional objectives) levels. Economic and financial indicators at national level are related to unit cost per patient and standard operational results. At regional level, these indicators are related to consumption, supplies and external service providers, personnel costs and purchases. Programme contract follow-up is provided by the RHA, with cross-monitoring (especially for the financial aspects) by the CAHS. RHA efficiency targets entail additional funding.

Performance-related incentives foster increasing service levels and a high level of resource utilization, as well as reducing inappropriate hospitalization. There are two types of incentive: institutional and internal (relating to services or professionals). The former are used for indicators such as re-hospitalization rates in the first five days; number of professionals involved in training programmes in the area of infection control; patients referred to the National Network for Continuing Care; outgoing patients in the specialties of internal medicine, general surgery and orthopaedics (specialties are adjusted according to the specificities of each institution); ambulatory surgery as a proportion of the total scheduled surgeries; or the average delay. They represent about 5% of the total financial resource contracted with each hospital (50% of it according to institutional objectives in the region, 30% according to national targets and 20% depending on regional objectives).

The setting up of internal incentives (when defined) largely depends on the management style of the AB (some may impose an incentives system, while others would prefer negotiating incentives with each service provider), but in any case prudent negotiation would be needed, taking into account the objectives defined in the programme contract and the guidelines of the Ministry of Finance and Ministry of Health. Hospitals do not have total autonomy to provide incentives as they please. Incentives are decided by the Ministries, with the intention of ensuring that hospitals do not compete with each other and that there is an integrated policy of incentives within the whole hospital sector.

Negative financial results remain within the hospital and are reflected in the hospital accounts (balance sheet and income statement). Currently, there are several hospitals with negative accumulated capitals. The successive accumulation of negative results can lead to technical bankruptcy (negative equity) of the hospital. This situation could be solved by a capital increase (because it is illegal directly to transfer capital for public enterprises without the necessary corresponding production) or by means of a convergence subsidy. However, it is a fixed value, defined a priori, and does not correspond to the total accumulated debt. There are no financial penalties as such in the programme contract, other than the risk that hospitals not meeting the contracted output levels would not receive all the funding. However, the methodology defined by the unit within the CAHS responsible for defining the methodology of the programme contract (Operational Unit for Finance and Contracting) defines penalties for marginal production (lower or upper); if in a "production line" the actual output is less than 50% of the contracted level, no payment at all will be made. Emergency units will still receive payments, albeit at a much lower price than contracted, in order to secure funding for fixed costs.

Hospital directors have limited autonomy to use existing capacity for raising funds (for example, from lending laboratory space to a nearby facility during nighttime hours or providing primary care in competition with private or public centres), as long as doing so would not undermine the full implementation of the programme contract. Hospitals could conceivably provide facilities to create an open primary health care consultation system using health centre resources. As providers of primary health care services, however, health centres are the entry point into the NHS and refer patients in need of specific services to public hospitals.

Based on this architectural articulation, it does not make sense for hospitals, in general, to provide primary care services other than under extreme circumstances. The NHS, in fact, foresees organizational models integrating both levels of care within the same structure – the "local health system". The agreement of the RHA and the approval of the Ministers of Health and Finance would be needed for substantive revenue-raising activities.

Aside from transfers from the state budget, public hospitals also generate revenue from payments for special services (for example, individual private rooms or other arrangements not provided for most users); from payments received from beneficiaries of the health subsystems or private insurance; and from flat-rate user charges for outpatient and diagnostic services (legally defined fees for certain services in emergency, surgery, outpatient and complementary health care fields). As already mentioned, ABs cannot set up co-payments. Further sources of revenue include private donations (especially for buying equipment and products from the users), and liabilities for infringing the rules of the organization relating to the operation of the system, and for using services and medical supplies fraudulently. As a whole, these payments account for as much as 15–20% of the overall hospital budget (Barros & de Almeida Simões, 2007).

The PEEH statute explicitly states that hospitals are obliged to raise the necessary money reserves, including legal reserves (not less than 20% of each period income in accordance with accounting standards) and reserves for investment (among others, a share of profits earned each year and revenue from contributions, endowments, grants, subsidies or any financial compensation to which the hospital is entitled).

11.3.3 Accountability arrangements

The PEEH statute explains that the AB may be dismissed because of a substantial deviation between the budget and its implementation a business deterioration including the quality of services provided and the non-fulfilment of the programme contract. Thus defined, the PEEH accountability framework includes the following main instruments:

- the report of the ABs;
- the report on the implementation of the multi-annual investment plan;
- the balance sheet and income statement, with specific elements appended;
- the statement of cash flows and ratio of loans to medium- and long-term finances; and
- the audit report, with the corresponding advisory report from the auditor – a distinction must be made here between the auditor and the internal auditor, the former being the body responsible for ensuring legality, regularity and sound hospital financial and asset management (appointed from among statutory/independent auditors or firms of statutory/independent chartered accountants)[34] and the latter carrying out internal control functions in areas relating to accounting, financial, operational, IT and human resources.[35]

This gives centre stage to the hospital monitoring system, including the definition of their own scorecard system. The AB is, in fact, responsible for defining such a system, and in principle has the autonomy to decide on the parameters for monitoring day-to-day activity. Financial accountability issues are dealt with by the General Inspectorate of Finance on a quarterly basis. Beyond that, however, true integrated hospital information systems are still the exception in Portugal, where standard reports alone add very little value to hospital organization or governance. Different subsystems deal with the areas

---

34 The financial statements are prepared on monthly basis by an accountant, usually on the hospital's staff. The auditor is responsible for auditing and certifying the annual and quarterly financial statements, in addition to acting upon requests from the AB relating to specific matters. As an external entity, it guarantees the legitimacy of the institution's accounts.

35 The internal auditor reports directly to the AB, auditing several areas and taking special care with regard to risk control, not only in support areas but also in clinical fields. S/he may also provide opinions on a diverse range of matters, at the request of the AB.

of human resources, various clinical activities, and so on, in a non-coordinated way. Notably even more absent is a common system for hospitals to report on their performance, aside from the accounting required for the programme contract monitoring reports.

All hospitals must now use the Official Accounting Plan of the Ministry of Health – although the system is still not mandatory and each hospital can choose its own implementation or system as long as it complies with the Official Accounting Plan. In the past, the Institute for Financial Management and Information (now the CAHS after the recent public administration reform) had developed a financial and accounting management system that was adopted by some hospitals. However, lack of integration with other information systems led to many hospitals dropping the application and using or developing one of their own. Only recently is computer software being introduced to generate robust management indicators, but most ABs are still involved in the learning process.

The PEEH statute allows greater intervention at the level of strategic trusteeship and oversight (exercised by the Ministries of Finance and Health) when required for the operation of all NHS institutions – both at operational level and at the level of economic rationality in terms of investment decisions. The Ministries have considerable capacity to review and reject, in terms of supervision at central and/or regional levels. This is embodied (regionally) by regular attendance of the AB sessions by a representative of the RHA, as well as (nationally) by cross-monitoring by CAHS, especially in the financial field. Municipal supervision – provided through a representative in the Advisory Council – is much less intense. This is all duly reflected by the work of the National Statistics Institute. The payer per se (the state) cannot suspend the contracted set of services defined in the programme contract; if significant deviations are detected, hospital governing bodies may first take corrective action, as recommended by the main shareholder (the state, through the Ministries of Finance and Health). This may include, in extreme cases, a unilateral suspension of programme contract elements (for example, when the production levels originally contracted are not met, indicating underperformance, the penalty could include a cut in the funding amount originally agreed).

In most cases the organization of the AB has followed ruling party guidelines, although during the first phase of public hospital corporatization, between 2002 and 2005, some municipalities appointed non-executive members. Unfortunately, the results of such practices were not optimal and non-executive members mainly acted as political commissaries, in some cases with total lack of health sector and hospital knowledge.[36] For a period after 2005, non-executive AB members ceased to be appointed, in response to proposals

---

36 In fact, the main complaint was that they brought political discussions with them into the AB.

from the municipality. Recently, non-executive members have begun to be appointed again by municipalities in which the governing political party differs from that of the national government. This was the case in Coimbra, where three of the largest Portuguese hospitals are located – the municipality proposed the appointment of non-executive members for each hospital (all of them physicians). The Ministries of Finance and Health, which ultimately makes the appointment, neglected to respond to this proposal. In light of the pre-2005 experience (and the related conclusions drawn), there is some concern about the possible consequences of these appointments.

In spite of official proclamations (the creation of an Advisory Council – with the mandate of assessing business plans, monitoring hospital activities and making recommendations for improving services to the population – is being contemplated, comprising a variety of actors[37]), citizens do not participate directly in decision-making, other than via the "suggestions box", the use of a "complaints book" (mandatory in all public and private institutions) and patient satisfaction surveys. Strictly speaking, Advisory Councils do not function well in practice, as noted in other studies (Raposo, 2007). No Board of Trustees is defined within the structure of PEEHs, with the hospital executive management role being exercised instead by the AB within the scope of the direct accountability relationships to the Ministries of Health and Finance, and other national and regional government entities.

In summary, PEEHs have rather limited decision-making capacity to enable them to adjust to unexpected trends, as well as little freedom from political intervention/interference. In most cases, the removal of ABs is due to political factors, normally a change in government(s). Recent reforms related to general public adminsistration introduced an Integrated Management and Performance Measurement in the Public Administration scheme[38] to be annually applied to the performance of public services, its directors and other employees, but as yet it is scarcely applied in the hospital sector. Aside from a very general principle of recognized merit, there are no explicit criteria for appointment of AB members beyond political trust, and examples of systematic assessment of AB performance in Portugal are indeed limited.

Preliminary steps towards the systematic evaluation of ABs are being taken by the Evaluation Committee of the PEEHs ABs, but the level of success is as yet unclear. The Evaluation Committee was created in 2008[39] with the task of

---

37 To include: a person of recognized merit appointed by the Ministry of Health; a representative of the municipality's PEEH headquarters, or, in the case of hospital centres, in each county in which their institutions are located, a representative of the RHA; a hospital users' representative; a representative elected by PEEH workers; a representative of service volunteering in PEEHs; and two actors – chosen by the AB of the PEEH – who are health care professionals but not tied to the hospital.

38 Law No. 66-B/2007.

39 Ordinance 3596/2008.

preparing the evaluation of the PEEH ABs, but the final report and proposed evaluation model for this Committee is not yet fully public (it was partly delivered at the end of 2008). More importantly, the evaluation of the ABs, anticipated to begin in 2009, has not been started. It was expected that this assessment would be linked with each hospital programme contract, but – according to outside observers – such as the Portuguese Observatory on Health Systems, the reason for the delay is mainly political in nature.[40] Bluntly put, it does not sound like an exaggeration to conclude that in reality ABs feel accountable first and foremost to the political authorities.

Some legislation has been published since 2007, strengthening hospital ABs' transparency and accountability, a summary of which is listed here.

- The new status of the public manager[41] strengthens and develops the system of incompatibilities, performance evaluation, payment calculations, definition of social security and compliance with applicable ethic rules, as well as good practices from international corporate governance and transparency examples. That is, the roles, functions and responsibilities of public managers become closer to those defined for managers in the private sector.

- Changes have been implemented in terms of the legal status of the state-owned companies sector and the public enterprises, to reflect on corporate governance issues.[42]

- The principles of good corporate governance in the state-owned companies sector[43] comprise a set of principles regarding the disclosure of information through a web site to be established by the DGTF,[44] as well as defining other, related elements.

- The Evaluation Committee has been created, the main objectives of which are to define and create an evaluation framework for hospital boards, and to implement this from 2008.

A result of the adoption of good governance principles is that all PEEHs should annually submit information to the DGTF to be published on its web site.

40 The NPM rules require the evaluation of public managers' performance. In their annual reports (Spring Report) greater dissemination of the information produced by this Committee is recommended, given its potential impact on hospital governance (OPSS, 2008, 2009). All the reports can be downloaded at the Portuguese Observatory on Health Systems web site (http://www.observaport.org (in Portuguese), accessed 2 May 2011).

41 Decree-law No. 71/2007.

42 Decree-law No. 300/2007.

43 Resolution of the Ministers' Council No. 49/2007.

44 Details are available on the web site of the DGTF (http://www.dgtf.pt/PresentationLayer/empresas.aspx?menuid=1060&exmenuid=1060 (in Portuguese), accessed 18 June 2011). See the DGTF web site for further information (http://www.dgtf.pt, accessed 18 June 2011). In particular:
• public information (corporate governance) regarding Public Enterprise Entities in the health care sector (http://www.dgtf.pt/SECTOR-EMPRESARIAL-DO-ESTADO-SEE/INFORMACAO-SOBRE-AS-EMPRESAS?menuid=1060&exmenuid=1060&temaid=28&sectorid=74, accessed 18 June 2011).

People will be able to access easily general and specific hospital information, as detailed here.

- General information, including members of the AB; economic performance; shareholder structure; assets; economic activity; financial situation; structure ratios; and other indicators.

- Organization-based information, including:
  - main characteristics: mission, objectives, company policies, the company's public service obligations, contractual terms of public service, the financing model underlying the provision of public service;
  - management guidelines;
  - governance model and governing bodies: position, name of the person occupying the position, election, term of mandate;
  - data relating to ABs: curriculum vitae, wages and other compensations, conflict of interests, functions and responsibilities of board members;
  - principles of good governance: internal and external hospital regulations; relevant transactions with related parties, other transactions; review of hospital sustainability in economic, social and environmental domains; assessment of compliance with principles of good governance and the code of ethics;
  - historical and current financial information: balance, income statement, statement of cash flows; and
  - public financial endeavours (capital transfers from state budget to hospital).

This information is to be updated on an annual basis, although not all hospitals will submit information to same level of detail. The only drawback, as already explained, relates to the Evaluation Committee, the results of which (namely, the evaluation of the ABs) have not yet been produced.

11.3.4 Operational governance: decision-making capacity versus responsibility

As already mentioned, each PEEH's AB is, in principle, free to decide its own allocation of resources (human, financial and material) in order to meet the objectives and targets defined in the programme contract. However, the effective capacity of the hospital and/or management team to implement decisions outside the clearly and formally defined corporate goals and objectives set at the political level (especially the ones negotiated in the programme contract) is strictly limited.

Some of the restrictions in the financial framework – including the need to obtain authorization from the responsible ministries to raise loans, transfer hospital services to other providers, and set up private clinical practices within the hospital – have already been discussed.

Another example is the need for regulation defining the hospital's internal organization to be approved by the responsible ministries, even if the PEEH statute in principle allows the AB autonomy to proceed. The autonomy to define authority and responsibility internally ("departmentalization", staff, committees and groups, decentralization, coordination systems, number and organization of the middle management, composition of different clinical committees and groups) is in practice curtailed by the requirement that clinical services should adhere to the Ministry of Health's planning of the hospital referral network – once again, anything departing from the centrally determined logic requires *ex ante* permission from the responnsible ministries.

In short, the operational governance of the hospitals does not include the capacity to find any short-cuts or alternative paths in the pursuit of hospital objectives. The current financial crisis has led to even stricter rules, further limiting the powers of ABs (relating to spending, hiring staff in the public sector, etc.).

Two areas in which the AB has somewhat greater autonomy include the setting up of clinical trials and the parameters for monitoring day-to-day activity.

1. The final decision regarding whether or not a new drug should be included in the hospital pharmacy (particularly relevant, for example, in the treatment of cancer patients) rests with the AB, with advice from the hospital Pharmaceutical and Therapeutics Commission, chaired by the clinical director (her/himself a member of the AB), but such drugs must previously have been included in the list approved by the National Authority of Medicines and Health Products. The participation of the hospital in clinical trials alone or in partnership is, however, a decision to be made solely by the AB; once chiefs of service or clinical staff make the proposal, the AB is responsible for accepting or declining those proposals and on what terms.

2. The AB also has total autonomy to decide on the parameters for monitoring day-to-day activity, including defining its own scorecard system, but progress has been rather patchy, with setbacks in terms of ensuring data compatibility, intra-system communication, database sharing, and so on. As already discussed, there is no common system across all hospitals, beyond that which is required in the reports for the monitoring of adherence to the programme contract. All the hospitals must use the Official Accounting Plan of the Ministry of Health.

An optimistic note is that hospitals have been investing heavily in the development of information systems in recent years in order to provide accurate and concise information, with different permission and detail levels defined for professionals' access. Information is now available in the vast majority of hospitals within the hospital intranet, and objectives of service teams are public and monitored. This aproach has two key objectives: first, to share data with clinicians, managers and other staff with the aim of improving collaborative work and more involvement in decision-making (where applicable); second (to a lesser extent, but increasingly important), to improve accountability and transparency within the organization, among professionals and groups. This latter objective clearly conflicts with the previous management approach modulated by centralized governance in health, entangled in a web of bureaucratic command-and-control systems.

Patients and the general public do not have access to the intranet, because it is focused on the internal needs of the organization. However, the information available to these hospitals (mainly through the sites of each of the PEEH hospitals,[45] the DGTF and the CAHS) is far greater than that available to traditional public hospitals. Aside from being used to improve transparency and accountability – through the provision of various documents (balance, income statement, quality reports, patient satisfaction studies, etc.) to all professionals – the intranet is used for collaborative working and sharing documents.

11.4 Conclusions

The structural reform of the Portuguese hospital sector, started in April 2002, attempted to corporatize hospitals and establish more viable, efficient centres for health care by merging existing hospitals – first transforming them into limited companies with exclusively public capital (*Hospitais SA*) and, later in 2005, transforming them into PEEHs. Such political choices are a vivid expression of the values of contemporary Portuguese society, combining concern and respect for individual and collective rights.

From a societal viewpoint, corporization was and continues to be seen as a facilitator and enabler of public hospital efficiency; the main emphasis in recent years has been on merging hospitals with different dimensions, capacities and specialties in order to make available resources hitherto underutilized. Policy focus on concentration has been strengthened by expanding corporatization to more hospitals and emphasizing quality improvement.

---

45 For more information on PEEHs, see the *Hospitais EPE* web site (http://www.hospitaisepe.min-saude.pt, accessed 18 June 2011).

Intuitively, corporatization has perhaps brought about more policy flexibility in terms of supply (stocks) and the hiring of human resources; there have also been improvements in the processes of billing and charging and refinements in contracting mechanisms (especially contract negotiation with units and professionals). It is probably fair to mention progress in business approaches, in planning and in management. In addition, there has been some increase in transparency and accountability, linked to information systems and related development of tools, both internally (intranet) and external (mainly through institutional web sites).

The truth, however, is that the lack of systematic collection and analysis of data and information simply precludes the drawing of final conclusions regarding whether or not the new models have contributed to performance improvement in areas such as health gain, equity, financial protection, patient responsiveness/satisfaction, clinical/outcomes, managerial proficiency, and so on, especially since 2005. Nevertheless, while not conclusive, some studies point to improvements in certain spheres, as detailed here.

- A study by the Evaluation Commission of Hospital Companies (*Hospitais SA*) (CAHSA, 2005a,b) addressed the areas of quality, access, production, cost, efficiency, supply, human resources and investment. In general, some increase in quantitative production and some efficiency gains were identified in terms of lower costs for similar outputs. In many dimensions, however, there were no apparent differences.

- A second study (Costa & Lopes, 2005) concluded that the corporatization process did not contribute to any decrease in access to health care, both in quantitative and qualitative terms, during the first two years, and even the extra production (surgical and medical) did not involve sacrifices in quality and efficiency of care.

- As part of the Court of Auditors monitoring programmes, a report that evaluated the hospital management model in the state sector from 2001 to 2004 concluded that adopting the new management model did not result in loss of efficiency. Quite the contrary, in fact, there is evidence of overall efficiency increases, clear statistical evidence of quality improvement in the group analysed and no evidence of losses of equity in terms of access (Court of Auditors, 2006).

- Finally, a 2008 Data Envelopment Analysis methodology study assessing the impact of the *Hospitais SA* management model on technical efficiency found such hospitals to be consistently the most efficient ones (Harfouche, 2008). It was noted, however, that the hospitals selected for corporatization already benefited from a higher level of technical efficiency than those not transformed at the time – so perhaps the process simply gave them further advantages for maximizing their efficiency under more flexible management rules.

Despite these positive aspects, the Portuguese Observatory on Health Systems considered this period to be a lost opportunity for several hospitals in some territories (OPSS, 2006). Having emerged in and developing within a persistent culture of centralized governance in health, entangled in a web of bureaucratic command-and-control systems imitated internally, those hospitals did not (know how to) implement or develop the necessary tools and negotiation models in which the new delegated powers would address responsibilities within a new framework. As already explained, political intervention continues to have too much emphasis on the formation of hospital ABs, especially in terms of their selection. Defining clear and objective criteria for AB membership – facilitating the setting up of effective teams and systematically evaluating AB performance – is rather urgent. Ascertaining the links between board performance and hospital results/outcomes is another important concern.

In summary, the hospital governance model – the topic of this chapter – remains a subject open to debate, as recognized by the Ministry of Health commission set up in 2010 to study the issue and propose possible alternatives.[46] To a certain extent, creating this commission was a way to recognize the failure of previous attempts and the need for urgent action. This is explicitly acknowledged in the fields of internal organization, management autonomy, clinical information systems, development of tools to measure and evaluate the integrated governance (both corporate and clinical), leadership, AB evaluation, training and recruitment, patient involvement, professionals' and services' internal incentive system development and services performance evaluation. The final report, available to the general public, ultimately points to the need for greater transparency and accountability, both external and internal. For example, the programme contract is followed on a regular basis by the RHA and the financial aspects are monitored by the CAHS. It is now argued that the contracts of the various internal units (departments), along with their indicators of production, quality, risk management, performance, incentives, training and research should be also publicly available (on the hospital web site), following approval by the AB.

Political will, implementation capacity and intelligent legislative measures are essential if a "culture of good governance" is to be created. It must also be recognized that it will take time to change traditional approaches.

---

46 Ordinance No. 10823/2010.

11.5 References

Barros P, de Almeida Simões J (2007). Portugal: health system review. *Health Systems in Transition*, 9(5):1–140.

CAHSA (2005a). *Resultados da Avaliação dos Hospitais SA – Sumário Executivo da Comissão de Avaliação dos Hospitais SA [Results from the assessment on the creation of enterprised hospitals – executive summary from the Evaluation Commission of Hospital Companies]*. Lisbon, Evaluation Commission of Hospital Companies.

CAHSA (2005b). *Resultados da Avaliação dos Hospitais SA – Sumário dos Resultados da Comissão de Avaliação dos Hospitais SA [Results from the assessment on the creation of enterprised hospitals, summary of main results from the Evaluation Commission of Hospital Companies]*. Lisbon, Evaluation Commission of Hospital Companies.

Costa C, Lopes S (2005). *Avaliação do desempenho dos hospitais SA – resultados provisórios [Performance evaluation of "Hospitais SA" – preliminary results]*. Lisbon, National School of Public Health.

Court of Auditors (2006). *Relatório de Auditoria no. 20/06: Relatório Global de Avaliação do Modelo de Gestão dos Hospitais do SEE (2001–2004) [Audit report no. 20/06: global assessment report of the management model of the hospitals of the state enterprise sector (2001–2004)]*. Lisbon, Court of Auditors.

Court of Auditors (2009). *Relatório no. 15/2009: Auditoria ao Programa de Parcerias Público Privadas da Saúde – Primeira vaga de Hospitais [Report no. 15/2009: audit program for public–private partnerships for health – first wave of hospitals]*. Lisbon, Court of Auditors.

Ferreira AS et al. (2010). A contratualização de cuidados de saúde [Healthcare contracting]. In: Simões J, ed. *30 Anos do Serviço Nacional de Saúde – um percurso comentado [30 years of the National Health Service – a route commented]*. Coimbra, Almedina:425–459.

Harfouche A (2008). *Hospitais Transformados em Empresas – Análise do Impacto na Eficiência: Estudo Comparativo [Hospitals transformed into enterprises – impact on efficiency analysis: a comparative study]*. Lisbon, Technical University of Lisbon Institute of Social and Political Sciences.

OPSS (2006). *Relatório de Primavera 2006 – Um ano de governação em Saúde: Sentidos e Significados [Spring report 2006 of the Portuguese Health System Observatory – a year of health governance: directions and interpreation]*. Lisbon, Portuguese Health System Observatory (http://www.observaport.org/node/119, accessed 22 December 2010).

OPSS (2008). *Relatório de Primavera 2008 – Sistema de Saúde Português: Riscos e Incertezas [Spring report 2008 of the Portuguese Health System Observatory – Portuguese health system: risks and uncertainties].* Lisbon, Portuguese Health System Observatory (http://www.observaport.org/rp2008, accessed 22 December 2010).

OPSS (2009). *Relatório de Primavera 2009 – 10/30 anos: Razões para continuar [Spring report 2009 of the Portuguese Health System Observatory – 10/30 years: reasons for continuing].* Lisbon, Portuguese Health System Observatory (http://www.observaport.org/rp2009, accessed 22 December 2010).

Raposo V (2007). *Governação hospitalar – uma proposta conceptual e metodológica para o caso português [Hospital governance – a conceptual and methodological proposal for the Portuguese case].* Coimbra, University of Coimbra Faculty of Economics.

11.6 Principal legislation

Law No. 48/90, 24 August 1990, Health Act (Fundamental Principles of Portuguese Health System).

Decree-law No. 558/99, 17 December 1999, establishes the legal regime of state-owned enterprises and public enterprises.

Law No. 27/2002, 8 November 2002, approves the new legal regime of hospital management and makes the first amendment to the Law no. 48/90.

Decree-law No. 233/2005, 29 December 2005, transform into public hospital enterprises (PEEH) the old hospital-companies (called *Hospitais SA*) and defines their statute.

Decree-Law No. 235/2006, 6 December 2006, establish the regime of installation, opening and functioning of pharmacy dispensing medications to the public inside the hospitals of the National Health Service and the conditions of their concession.

Decree-law No. 71/2007, 27 March 2007, approves the new status of public manager.

Resolution from the Ministers Council no. 49/2007, 28 March 2007, approves the principles of good corporate governance of state-owned enterprises.

Decree-law No. 300/2007, 23 August 2007, changes the legal regime of state-owned enterprises and public enterprises.

Law 66-B/2007, 28 December 2007, establishes the integrated management and performance measurement in public administration.

Ordinance No. 3596/2008, 16 January 2008, creates the Evaluation Committee of the Administration Boards of PEE hospitals.

Ordinance No. 10823/2010, 1 July 2010, creates and define the composition of the Technical Group for the Reform of the Internal Organization of Hospitals.

Chapter 12
Spain

Arturo A. Álvarez and Antonio Durán

12.1 The unexpected birth of new governance arrangements in Spain

The Spanish National Health System (*Sistema Nacional de Salud*, SNS) offers universal health care coverage for all residents in Spain and provides publicly funded health services, mainly financed through taxation at national level. Publicly funded health services are, in general, free at the point of use and responsibility for their organization largely rests with the 17 regions or *comunidades autónomas* (ACs) (García-Armesto et al., 2010).

Since the early 1990s, Spain has explored new hospital governance arrangements. It has done so while decentralizing hospital management via ad hoc, last-minute politically driven legislation, which has resulted in a rather confusing, fragmented regulatory framework, with various national and regional norms superseding each other. Yet, this section will sustain the thesis that such development – the result of a highly political process in the highly political environment of post-Franco politics in Spain – has opened the way for innovative governance approaches.

12.1.1 Birth of the Spanish SNS

Evolving from a bureaucratic, centralized, resource-scarce and fragmented system funded by social insurance contributions, the current tax-funded SNS in Spain provides (almost) comprehensive coverage to (virtually) all residents, (essentially) free at the point of use. These principles were included in the 1978 Spanish Constitution after Franco's death.

Political transition to democracy came about alongside political devolution to the ACs. A few ACs (Cataluña, País Vasco, Navarra, Galicia and Andalucía) were soon allocated powers to develop their own regional health policies with the INSALUD, established in 1978 as the SNS executive, responsible for managing the health care system in those regions without devolved power. Each AC established over the years their health executives to run their own regional health system; when authority for health care was transferred to all ACs in 2002, the INSALUD was abolished (Durán, Lara & van Waveren, 2006).

ACs, however, copied the inherited bureaucratic model of the national public administration, resulting in heavily centralized and politicized administrative structures (Ballart & Ramió, 2000); devolution to the regional level did not translate further down the scale to the local levels.

An additional systemic change of the Spanish health system involved ideas and practices from the NPM paradigm (Hood, 1991), which was fashionable around the world in the 1980s and led to a number of changes in the Spanish public administration (Gallego Calderón, 2002). In this context, public management attracted the attention of some national policy-makers, civil servants and an enthusiastic group of managers within the new SNS, who sought to modernize the management of hospitals and health care centres. It is now clear, however, that the first wave of modernization lacked strategic vision and political support, and innovations had only limited impact (Belenes, 2003). The detachment in 1981 of the Ministry of Health and Consumer Affairs from the Ministry of Labour and Social Security also paved the way for more in-depth reforms in the mid-1980s.

The 1986 General Healthcare Law (*Ley 14/1986, de 25 de abril, General de Sanidad*) sought to integrate the various health care structures and to coordinate levels of care. In article 67, the possibility of establishing partnerships with the private sector was even considered. However, the Law did not address alternative management models for the SNS, which retained many features of the old administrative model, especially a statutory position for health care staff (currently regulated by the Law on the Framework Statute of Health Personnel (*Ley 55/2003, de 16 de diciembre, del Estatuto Marco del Personal Sanitario de los Servicios de Salud*), which ensured that salaries remained not related to performance (Martín & López del Amo, 2003)).

Some of the relevant NPM *tools* were by then already being gradually incorporated in the system without resistance, and continued to do so. For example, health *targets* started to be used at regional level even before the 1986 General Healthcare Law (which referred generically to them in articles 43 and 54), although there never was a nationwide health target strategy (Alvarez-

Dardet, 2002). There were also Consortia (*Consortia*) in some parts of Spain (specifically Catalonia) which were run along slightly different lines compared with regular public health care centres.

In 1991, that is, only five years after approving what was supposed to be the backbone, enduring health law of the democratic period, the parliament sponsored a Commission for the Analysis and Evaluation of the SNS (*Comisión de Análisis y Evaluación del SNS*, known as *Comisión Abril* after its chairman, the former centre-right Minister Abril Martorell, one of the architects of the political transition after Franco). Administrative rigidity, excessive centralization and staff apathy were identified as specific problems by the Commission, which made 64 suggestions for modernizing the SNS, with a purchaser–provider split and the adoption of new management tools among them (Gómez de Hita, 2000). Proposals from the Commission encountered great opposition from unions and other health care groups (Guillén & Cabiedes, 1998).

In that context, "managerial" improvements continued under their own steam. In 1991, a Minimum Basic Data Set (*Conjunto Mínimo Básico de Datos*) was introduced to codify hospital discharges. In 1994, INSALUD started using "programme contracts" (*contratos-programa*) with hospitals, as a mechanism to promote activity planning within those hospitals and make more explicit the link between funding and performance (Martín, 1996). Retrospective payment systems for hospital activity were – at least formally – replaced around 1997 by prospective budgets based on DRGs and supported by different accounting tools. DRGs were first piloted in 18 public hospitals and, after evaluation, they were "supported" in the following years by national and regional health authorities (García-Cornejo, 2008).

12.1.2 Altering the original hospital plans

Within this "tradition" of initial tentative innovation in the regions, a particular law was issued – partly or wholly accepted by the central administration – regulating the above-mentioned Consortia (*Ley 30/1992, de 26 de noviembre, de Régimen Jurídico de las Administraciones Públicas y del Procedimiento Administrativo Común*). This law complemented a previous one (Law 7/1985 on the same matter – *Ley 7/1985, de 2 de abril, Reguladora de las Bases de Régimen Local*) and opened the way to merging resources from several administrations, so that a more efficient use of resources could be made. For the first time, the need for pragmatic arrangements in the field of hospital governance was expressed.

Somehow signalling an identity of its own, while emphasizing the opposition to its main rival's policies, the Government of Andalucía (ruled by the Socialist Party) subscribed to a model of hospital governance named the *Empresa Pública*

Sanitaria (Public Healthcare Company) in 1993, and the *Empresa Pública Hospital Costa del Sol* was established in Marbella, a tourist city (*Disposición adicional Decimoctava de la Ley 4/1992, de 30 de diciembre, de Presupuestos de la Comunidad Autónoma de Andalucía para 1993*; statutes approved by the *Decreto 104/1993, de 3 de agosto, por el que se constituye la empresa pública Hospital de la Costa del Sol y se aprueban sus estatutos*).

Another key development took place in 1994, in terms of regulating the "Foundations model" (*Fundaciones, Ley 30/1994, de 24 de noviembre, de Fundaciones y de incentivos fiscales a la participación privada en actividades de interés general*). While this norm applied to the establishment and functioning of foundations in all sectors, it was particularly sought by health policy-makers to bring into play more flexible organizational arrangements alongside the separation of purchasing and provider functions that the INSALUD was (timidly) introducing (Ferrándiz Manjavacas, 1999). Later, in 2002 (as already indicated, the year when the process of devolving health power to the regions was completed and the INSALUD was abolished), an updated Foundations Law (*Ley 50/2002, de 26 de diciembre, de Fundaciones*) was issued to replace Law 30/1994.

In 1996, with the conservative Partido Popular (PP) for the first time in power at national level after 14 consecutive years of socialist governments, legislation was introduced explicitly promoting new types of hospital governance. The Royal Law-Decree (*Real Decreto-ley 10/1996, 17 de junio, sobre habilitación de nuevas formas de gestión del Sistema Nacional de Salud*) allowed for the use of various governance models for managing the INSALUD hospitals, including Consortia, Foundations and so on. Notably, the use of the legal tool *Real Decreto Ley* – in principle only recommended for fast-tracking legislation through parliament under exceptional/urgent circumstances – was justified "based on the need to set up a new governance model before pilot hospitals were built" (*Real Decreto-ley 10/1996*, p. 424). This exceptional mechanism was later on duly replaced, in terms of its essential components, by a more conventionally produced law (*Ley 15/1997, de 25 de abril, de habilitación de nuevas formas de gestión del Sistema Nacional de Salud*).

With the explicit aim to "introduce more flexible mechanisms for managing statutory hospital staff", the government of the day tried to promote a Parliamentary Agreement for the Reform and Modernization of the NHS (*Acuerdo Parlamentario para la Reforma y Modernización del SNS*, Diciembre 1997), but failed (Freire, 1998). It then created the "Public Healthcare Foundations" model by promulgating at the very last minute a law with the most peculiar title of "*Law on Fiscal, Administrative and Social Measures*" (*Ley 50/1998, de 30 de diciembre, de Medidas Fiscales, Administrativas y del Orden*

Social) annexed to the General Budget Law (*Ley 49/1998, de 30 de diciembre, de Acompañamiento a los Presupuestos del Estado*). It was also a remarkable move in another way: Law 30/1994 on Foundations was fully available and could have been enforced immediately to transform staff into non-statutory, ordinarily contracted workers, but – probably due to the fear of conflict with the militant trade unions – a new model was created instead, retaining the statutory status (permanent jobs) of the existing health care staff.

In 1999, the AC of Valencia – also governed by the conservatives – granted to a private group of companies (by means of an "administrative concession" (*concesión administrativa*)) the right to run the public hospital in Alzira, making use of the opportunities presented by Law 15/1997 (and the 1995 Procurement Law – *Ley 13/1995 de 18 de mayo, de Contratos de las Administraciones Públicas*) (Marín Ferrer, de Rosa & Gómez Gómez, 2003; Marín Ferrer & de Rosa Torner, 2007). This was the first instance of such an openly pro-business concession and initiated a vivid discussion within the Spanish health care community.

Soon afterwards, Royal Decree 29/2000 (*Real Decreto 29/2000, de 14 de enero, sobre nuevas formas de gestión del Instituto Nacional de la Salud*) listed the existing types of hospital self-governance models, including Public Healthcare Foundations, Consortia and Foundations. This norm confirmed the management autonomy of these entities, while preserving and guaranteeing their public service through controls and mechanisms implemented to ensure the observance of constitutional principles, as well as coordination and cooperation between health centres.

After another political change at central level in 2004, the new government ruled out any attempt to homogenize the situation in the various regions (the slogan for its political alliances with the nationalists was *España plural*, meaning "plural Spain"). At the same time, the 2007 Public Sector Procurement Law (*Ley 30/2007, de 30 de octubre, de Contratos del Sector Público*) attempted to narrow the autonomy of most new governance initiatives designed in the previous period. The debate regarding the real value of hospital management innovative experiences entered the parliament in 2008 through the Parliamentary Health Committee (*Comisión de Sanidad del Congreso de los Diputados*), but no clear conclusion was reached.

At the end of 2010, the possibility of developing a Health Pact (*Pacto por la Sanidad*) was discussed, seeking the agreement of all parliamentary parties on key founding principles of the SNS. A number of key goals relating to the basket of services to be provided by the SNS, the level of health expenditure required to make the system sustainable, the expected quality levels to be guaranteed, and so on, were also included, as well as hospital governance and new management models – no longer as a technical issue, but rather as part of the political agenda. It is worth noting that new approaches in the AC of Madrid, for example, faced rather strong opposition, with those opposing the health pact claiming that they would just lead to the privatization of the public health care system. The approval of the health pact, which seemed on the cusp of being signed immediately – was then postponed "at least until 2013", after the upcoming round of local, regional and national elections.

12.2 Five self-governed hospital types in Spain

The previous section explained how a genuinely enthusiastic, pro-democracy political change brought about (almost silently) some five "different models" of self-governed hospitals, coexisting with both typically public and typically private hospital management arrangements (Sánchez Caro, 2000; Menéndez Rexach, 2008). Table 12.1 provides a summary of the legal status of the five models of self-governed hospitals in Spain.

Table 12.1 *Self-governed hospital types in Spain and their legal status*

Type of legal entity	Service delivery modality	Regulation modality	Precise legal framework
Public Healthcare Company (public law entity)	Direct (public sector coverage and delivery)	Legal personality as public sector entity but resource use and management according to private law	• Specific law by Andalusian Parliament (*Disposición Adicional 18 de* Law 4/1992 *de Presupuestos de la Comunidad Autónoma de Andalucía*) • The national law that regulates these public entities is Law 30/1992 • Statutes by Decree 104/1993 • Staff under private employment law (Workers Statute – *Estatuto de los Trabajadores*) but possible civil service or statutory law • Public Sector Procurement Law (material resources management and contracting of goods and services) • Public Sector Budget Law (financing and budgetary management); control by auditing
Public Healthcare Foundation (state-owned foundation)	Direct (public sector coverage and delivery)	Entity with legal personality of its own, created by public and/or not-for-profit persons and with its own assets ascribed to "general interest" goals	• Law 50/1998 • Specific statutes • Statutory staff • Civil law for goods and services contracts

Type of legal entity	Service delivery modality	Regulation modality	Precise legal framework
Foundation	Direct (public sector coverage and delivery)	Entity with legal personality of its own, created by public and/or not-for-profit persons and with its own assets ascribed to "general interest" goals	• Law 50/2002 (to replace Law 30/1994) • Specific statutes • Staff under private employment law (with own agreement "*convenio propio*") • Civil law for goods and services contracts
Consortium	Direct (public sector coverage and delivery)	Entity with legal personality and assets of its own, created by several public administrations and/or not-for-profit private entities	• Law 30/1992 (complementing Law 7/1985) • Specific statutes • Staff under private employment law (Workers Statute – *Estatuto de los Trabajadores*) • Contracts for goods and services: public sector procurement law • Financial control by means of audits
Administrative Concession	Mixed, indirect (public sector coverage and private sector delivery)	Hospital building and running by means of concession. Both primary health care and specialized care included	• Law 15/1997 (and Law 13/1995 *Administraciones Públicas*) • Public tender: terms of reference (*pliego de condiciones*) • 70% staff under private employment law + specific collective working agreement) and 30% statutory staff • Fully fledged private law

In order to further assess each model's characteristics, the authors of this chapter contacted various CEOs and Presidents of the Boards of Trustees – one representative of each of the above governance modalities. The main selection criteria across the country were (1) that the hospital concerned was the first one adopting such a managerial model; (2) "popularity" – meaning that the hospital was well known and usually mentioned among commentators when discussing this issue; (3) similarity of size (four of the hospitals provide services in an area with about 245 000 people); and (4) availability of information about the hospital on the Internet, in publications, and so on. The findings are detailed in the subsections that follow.

12.2.1 The Public Healthcare Company[47]

The first and most remarkable example of a Public Healthcare Company is the *Hospital Costa del Sol* in Marbella (Andalucía). In 1993, the government of this region (with a population of 8 million) introduced this model, with the

---

47 Authors' own translation.

declared purpose of granting more managerial freedom to hospital managers. The brand new *Hospital Costa del Sol* thus became an enterprise regulated by private law (*empresa*). In subsequent years, additional examples of this model in the same region have included the *Hospital de Poniente*, the *Hospital Alto Guadalquivir* and the *Empresa Pública de Emergencias Sanitarias* (in charge of all emergencies in Andalucía). The *Hospital de Fuenlabrada* in Madrid is also a Public Healthcare Company.

The main feature of Public Healthcare Companies is that health care professionals are non-statutory staff (*contratados laborales*) instead of civil servants. They are consequently regulated by the common Workers Statute (*Estatuto de los Trabajadores*) and related legislation. There is a performance-related salary scheme for the clinical staff. Both changes were expected to lead to more productivity, better quality of care and higher patient and worker satisfaction. Some available results seem to confirm this as being the case, but traditionally run top hospitals in the region continued to perform better in certain fields (perceived quality, average waiting time for selected procedures, selected unit costs, and so on).

In spite of such ambitious intent, however, exhaustive control by public authorities seems to have been the main driver of Public Healthcare Companies. At present, for example, although the Board of Governors (*Consejo de Administración*) is legally expected to oversee the functioning of the hospital, in practice it seems to have been far more active in controlling the finances than in developing business strategies or innovative planning. Upwards accountability from the CEO seems to be rather ad hoc. In addition, Public Healthcare Company hospitals suffer from three annual inspections: from an external auditing company; from the auditing unit of the regional government (*Intervención*) and from the *Cámara de Cuentas* of the Andalusian Parliament, respectively – all requiring basically the same paperwork.

The hospitals' budget has been approved annually from the start by the regional parliament (each Public Healthcare Company in fact, has its own annual budget within the overall budget of the regional government). However, although the hospitals' leadership prepared this as a prospective budget, according to both population size and needs, representatives of the Andalucian Regional Finance Department (*Consejería de Hacienda*) at the Board of Governors have always opposed any budget increase in line with increases in the reference population or the expansion of services provided. In fact, they have imposed funding increases no larger than 2–3% per year, similar to increases granted to virtually all other hospitals in the region.

In 1996 the Regional Finance Department prohibited the hospitals from making use of any profit – including for reinvestment in facility improvement or the purchase of any new technology: any net profit the hospital achieved at the end of the fiscal year should simply be returned to the Regional Finance Department. In fact, the Public Healthcare Companies recently seem to have lost financial autonomy almost completely. While originally, for example, they were not obliged to abide by the Public Sector Procurement Law, they have now been included under such regulation, which leaves little room to negotiate prices with providers, and so on.

Since 2008 (according to article 27 of *Ley 3/2008 de 23 de diciembre, del Presupuesto de la Comunidad Autónoma de Andalucía para el año 2009*) any new post to be advertised in any Andalusian public hospital (including the Public Healthcare Company hospital) must be approved by the Regional Finance Department and the Regional Department of Justice (*Consejería de Justicia*). Both departments review the profile of the position before it is advertised, although they do not become involved in the actual process of candidate selection.

12.2.2 The Public Healthcare Foundation

The most prominent example of the Public Healthcare Foundation model is the *Hospital del Oriente de Asturias "Francisco Grande Covián"* in the north of Spain, although the hospital was originally established as a foundation in 1997, barely six years after the establishment of the first Public Healthcare Companies. It became a Public Healthcare Foundation after opposition parties won control of regional government in the 2008 elections, signalling a political change. The *Hospital de Inca* in the Balearic Islands is another example of this model.

Like the Public Healthcare Company, the Public Healthcare Foundation is a public entity but the key difference between them is that the latter model is staffed by statutory personnel. Usually, the governing body is also a Board of Governors with representatives of the regional health department and the local authority, and responsible for appointing the hospital CEO.

Public Healthcare Foundations were described at the time as "the most radical change that has ever taken place in Spanish public hospitals" (Freire, 1999) but the results of this initiative (as differing from ordinary public sector management) seem to be much more disappointing than those of the Public Healthcare Companies. It is probably worth mentioning also that after repeatedly contacting both above hospitals we have been unable to properly interview any manager representing this model (in fact, the CEO of the *Hospital de Inca* argued a "need of prior authorization to speak to us" and referred us to the regional health department for obtaining such permit. We interpreted this as a self-evident (negative) indicator of autonomy, and decided not to proceed further).

12.2.3 The Foundation

The Foundations Law (Law 30/1994) established the model of Foundations to run public hospitals. The *Hospital Universitario Fundación Alcorcón* (Madrid) is an important example, well known among United Kingdom health commentators, since the former Secretary of State for Health Alan Milburn visited it in 2001 and was allegedly inspired to set up the English Foundation Trust's model. Other examples of the Foundation model include the *Hospital de Manacor* in the Balearic Islands and some hospitals in Galicia (Barbanza, Virxe da Xunqueira, Verín and Salnés – although their Foundation status was abolished in July 2008 by a left-wing coalition government, reverting to the traditional model of hospital governance).

A Foundation is a non-profit-making organization regulated by private law, which means that the Public Sector Procurement Law related to "harmonized contracts (*contratos armonizados*) only marginally applies to them. Hospital activity is agreed by means of an annual contract with the regional health authority, with the main objectives tending to fit those of the regional health system programme contract.

The Foundations employ non-statutory health care professional staff using performance-related payment schemes, usually up to a 10% of total earnings. They operate more autonomously than the previous two models discussed, with the capacity, for example, to decide the basket of services to be provided (although, in practice, agreement with the regional health authority tends to have been previously sought). Foundations are also free to provide services to patients covered by private health insurance and even fully private patients, discretionarily. Importantly, their non-profit-making nature means that all possible profits need to be reinvested in the hospital.

Foundations are free to manage their own cash flow and to pay their providers directly, on either a monthly or bi-monthly basis, which allows them to negotiate better deals; they also have the autonomy to choose where to invest and whether to rent or buy their equipment. The only financial requirement the Foundation needs to meet is not going below 20% of the original capital; within that context, maintaining the hospital patrimony (the property/real estate) is, therefore, subject to achieving the goals established in the regulatory statutes governing the hospitals.

The governance body of a Foundation is its Board of Trustees/Governors (*Patronato*), on which public institutions, such as the town hall, local university and similar institutions may sit. By law this body is only obliged to meet twice per year, so its control is at arm's length and upward accountability from the management is rather weak. Experience shows that the regional health authorities often engage with the Foundation management as much as they do with any other public hospital.

As explained regarding the Public Healthcare Company, control of the Foundations seems to be heavily bureaucratic; the hospital interviewed, for example, also undergoes three annual inspections (from an external auditing company, from the auditing unit of the regional health authority and from the *Tribunal de Cuentas* of the Madrid regional Parliament).

It is worth mentioning again that the updated Foundations Law (Law 50/2002) – issued to replace Law 30/1994 – had the stated purposes of easing the rigid control mechanisms and reforming the organization of the Board of Trustees/Governors. The law was rhetorically presented as *an effort to incorporate innovative experiences with administrative law taking place in other countries*, but it is unclear at this stage whether those goals have been achieved, as illustrated by increasing control on the part of the politicians and the aforementioned conversion of some Foundations into Public Healthcare Foundations.

12.2.4 The Consortium

Probably best represented in Spain by the *Consorci Sanitari del Maresme* (Cataluña), one of the biggest in Spain (established in 1998 to replace a previous *consorcio* functioning for almost a decade), a Consortium hospital is a legal figure resulting from merging resources from several public authorities, usually the regional government and a lower local authority (*ayuntamiento y/o comarca*). Most examples of this model are located in Cataluña, such as the *Consorcio Sanitario Integral de Cataluña*, the *Consorcio de Vic* and the *Consorcio de Tarrasa*. In Andalucía, a *Consorcio Sanitario Público del Aljarafe (Hospital San Juan de Dios)* has recently been established in Seville.

The Consortia employ non-statutory health care professionals as staff and offer them performance-related incentives amounting to 8–10% of their income. They agree an annual contract with the regional health authority (for example, *Catsalut* in Cataluña or *SAS* in Andalucía) in line with the broad objectives of the programme contract, which the latter signs with hospitals providing services to publicly covered patients. *Catsalut* used to pay hospitals according to activity, but recently this was changed to a mixed system of capitation and activity-based payment.

The Consortia have real autonomy to decide on the basket of services they wish to offer, often supplementing the public basket with extra services in dental care, maxillofacial surgery, natural therapies, and so on – although in practice they agree such service expansion with the regional health authority. In other words, they also provide services to patients covered by private health insurance (about 5–6% of their income) and treat fully private patients, usually restricted to ambulatory care. They also have the autonomy to decide whether to rent or buy equipment.

For these reasons, Consortia are only subject to the Public Sector Procurement Law in terms of a limited set of issues and quantities, being allowed to outsource ("externalize") most support activities. The shared and agreed financial requirement to ensure the sustainability of the hospital is to break even, but Consortia remain free from having to return the benefits to the hospital (neither are they obliged to return the money to the regional government).

Consortia also have the autonomy to choose where to invest, but subject to (in the case of significant volumes) discussions with and approval by the regional health authority. The process starts with the CEO elevating the investment plan proposal to the Board of Governors (*Consejo Rector*), which includes regional health authority and local authority representatives and meets monthly. In addition to overseeing the functioning of the Consortium, the Board is responsible for: approving the business plan and the budget, approving investment decisions, creating new posts, appointing managers and approving the contract with the regional health authority. This Board also holds the CEO accountable for day-to-day hospital management, and monitors quality, activity, financial position, waiting lists, and so on. It formulates any proposal to change hospital norms (*estatutos*), but the regional health authority makes the final decision in such matters.

Hospital managers are free to reorganize posts and functions, with the prior approval of the Board of Governors. Each hospital has the right to design its own health information system. Data on waiting lists must be sent to the regional health authority on a monthly basis and quarterly updates on the financial situation of the hospital must be sent to the auditing unit of the regional government.

As mentioned in previous examples, the hospital undergoes annually three inspections (from an external auditing company, from the auditing unit of the regional government (*Intervención*) and from the Auditor's Office (*Sindicatura de Cuentas*) in the case of the Catalan Parliament.

12.2.5 The Administrative Concession

By means of the *concesión administrativa*, a private concessionary company (in Spain, usually a joint venture between private health insurers, health groups, building societies or banks) is given the right to build a hospital and provide health care services to a defined population, usually for 10 years, with the possibility of extending it for a further 5 years. The first and best-known administrative concession hospital is the *Hospital de la Ribera* in Alzira (Valencia), which at present integrates primary and specialized care (Marín Ferrer, de Rosa & Gómez Gómez, 2003; Marín Ferrer & de Rosa Torner, 2007). Following the Alzira initiative, this region established other hospitals under the same management model: the *Hospital de Torrevieja*, the *Hospital Marina Alta de Denia*, the *Hospital de Manises* and the *Hospital de Vinalopó* in Elche. The AC of Madrid has also established one administrative concession, the *Hospital Infanta Elena* in Valdemoro.

Differing from most other PFIs, for example in the United Kingdom, administrative concession hospitals in Spain are managed by the concessionary company, but funding is provided from public sources. The Madrid region has just built seven new hospitals, in Majadahonda, San Sebastián de los Reyes, Coslada, Madrid-Vallecas, Aranjuez, Arganda del Rey, and Parla – all are PFIs in terms of composition of the hospitals, but do not include management or provision of services.

The funding formula for these hospitals is capitation (although a number of items are currently excluded, such as oxygenotherapy, transport, outpatient pharmaceuticals, prostheses, etc.). In 2011, the capitation fee for the Valencia concessions was €607.14. In the context of patient choice, administrative concession hospitals must cover the treatment costs of people from within their catchment area who are treated elsewhere at 100% rate, but are only reimbursed 80–85% of costs for health services provided to patients from any other area.

Although alignments with the overall objectives of the regional programme contracts always exist, administrative concession hospitals are in themselves not fully linked to the regional hospital programme contracts, and may negotiate their own contracts with the regional health departments (*acuerdo de gestión*). The hospitals are also free to decide on their own sources of capital investment for large items of new equipment, renovations, and so on (including bank loans), as well as the sources of operating capital for regular day-to-day expenses.

The CEO can, in turn, decide on specific financial arrangements for any given piece of equipment, as well as proposing increases in the basket of services provided and contracting out services, if required. The only pre-established requirement with which the hospital should comply is that there is a limit to the "authorized" profit rate, capped at 7.5% over the whole concession period (any additional profit after taxes must be reimbursed to the regional health authority).

Administrative concession hospitals operate according to a rigid accountability arrangement and strict controls preclude the hospital from selecting risks and patients. Day-to-day control is exercised by a regional health ministry delegate (*Comisionado de la Consejeria de Sanidad*) based at the hospital, supported by a number of units (information, quality control, finance, etc.) directly under her/his command and with the capacity to control, inspect and sanction. This arrangement ensures her/his full access to information regarding hospital activity, patient satisfaction, financial performance, and so on. Approving the treatment of patients who do not belong to the primary care district, as well as later ensuring accurate billing for the services provided to them, are critical responsibilities of the *Comisionado*.

In the case of the *Hospital de la Ribera de Alzira*, statutory staff were given a choice between being transferred to a non-statutory scheme or retaining their statutory status. About 30% of the existing personnel refused to change, so around 70% of the administrative concession hospital staff are non-statutory and the other 30% are statutory. After this, all new staff automatically become non-statutory. The hospital is entitled to contract new staff without using the *regional employment list* (an official job-seekers list). Both groups of staff, in fact, have separate management lines – the non-statutory personnel are managed by the hospital CEO, while the *Comisionado* manages the statutory staff. Likewise, statutory and non-statutory staff have different incentive schemes; incentives for non-statutory staff are agreed with the unions.

The hospital CEO is appointed and removed by the concessionary company – in fact, the CEO's contract is signed by the representative (*apoderado general*) of the company, although approval of the regional health department is required. A second layer of accountability is provided by the Joint Commission (*Comisión Mixta*) between the company and the regional health authority, which meets three times per year. The CEO is also accountable to the concessionary company shareholders, usually through a joint shareholder/CEO committee, which meets monthly.

IT plays a major role in the governance of the hospital. The regional health ministry has access to hospital data in order to assess clinical quality, activity and finances on a regular basis. Administrative concession hospitals undergo annually two main inspections: from an external auditing company and from the auditing unit of the regional government.

12.3 Discussion

The five "models" described in some detail in this chapter configure (in our opinion) a kind of continuum in terms of self-governance, as follows: the Public Healthcare Company (1), is less autonomous than the Public Healthcare Foundation (2), which is less autonomous, in turn, than the Foundation (3), the Consortium (4) and the Administrative Concession (5). In the extremes, the rather top-down managed Public Healthcare Company is just a slight deviation from the traditional publicly owned, publicly managed hospital, while the more autonomous administrative concession hospital sometimes behaves like a commercial company, with only loose ties with the public sector owner-cum-funder.

The surveyed strategic and operational dimensions of the proposed framework seem to be relevant for assessing the level of hospital autonomy in Spain. Within such a framework, the key analytical dimensions that best seem to reveal whether each of these hospital types has the autonomy that they are supposed to enjoy, in our understanding, are those listed here.

- The ability to contract out services with providers and health care staff. In Spain, the key difference seems to be whether and to what extent the hospital is bound to the stringent Public Sector Procurement Law.

- The different accountability arrangements that exist. The more arm's-length, the stronger and more efficient the accountability arrangements seem to be. The accountability structures of the administrative concession model seem to be relatively effective in holding managers to account (in particular, through the ability of the regional health department to directly access hospital information), although the role and ability of the Commissioner raises questions about cooptation by the provider. Since inspection and control requirements in Spain entail perhaps too much bureaucracy at present, a consistent single auditing scheme could add value – excess (futile) control as opposed to accountability seems to be a problem in all hospital models.

- The status of the workforce (whether they are statutory staff, contracted, etc.) is also relevant, but probably less so than originally understood.

- One plausible explanation regarding why new governance schemes have (almost) exclusively been applied to newly built hospitals is the opposition of trade unions, and politicians' fear of clashing with them. The experiences in Valencia (Alzira and others) and Madrid illustrate both the feasibility of introducing those changes whenever the political will exists, and also the need to do so by means of (for example) parallel managerial lines, according to staff working and legal conditions (both statutory and non-statutory); that is, a give-and-take approach and trade-offs.

Paradoxically enough, the coincidence of two highly polarized political parties "going beyond the written norm" only five years after the joint approval of a core general health law is highly revealing. Furthermore, we believe that such abundance of nuances attests in the Spanish context to the substantially unplanned nature of the developments. In other words, beyond resulting in a fragmented regulatory framework with various national and regional norms (see Table 12.1), the fact that all five Spanish models of hospital self-governance have been established by last-minute, ad hoc, politically driven legislation shows that innovative governance arrangements do not necessarily require conscientious planning exercises – something found in other areas, as shown in the first two chapters of this book.

Some of the innovative features of hospital self-governance models in Spain have lately been eroded by strong centralizing forces at regional level (this has proved to be the case for Public Healthcare Companies and Public Healthcare Foundations in particular; the room for manoeuvring for these has gradually been reduced since they were first established by the health authorities concerned). In our understanding, this is only an expression of the highly dynamic nature of these changes in the politically overloaded environment of present-day Spain (one more indication that the wider institutional context beyond the specific health sector arrangements also affects and determines the true autonomy of individual hospitals). Hospital autonomy, in other words, is not a specific, encapsulated feature of the health field but rather responds to broader political and social characteristics.

While confirming the idea that autonomy is a key dimension of governance, our study highlights the limitations of either the macro, purely political level or the meso- and micro-level management domains in fully explaining what is happening in many Spanish health system and health care settings. Such changes would be better addressed not through the concept of management but through the concept of governance, as defined in the first half of this book: that is, changes in the methods and the tools used to govern the public sector – away from command-and-control systems, public administration or management-focused models – in response to changes in state–society relationships currently transforming social structures, policy processes, political systems and institutions, organizational arrangements, and so on.

In summary, the various "models" of self-governing hospitals tried so far in Spain, and the up-and-down, forward-and-backward steps within each model show that, far from being simple technical solutions, innovative governance models become embedded in powerful political and social structures, which can either limit or enhance their capacity for change. In other words, context and politics matter.

In broader and more important terms, the very description of the above-mentioned models illustrates the limitations of traditional managerial arrangements for solving the problems of a rapidly changing western society such as Spain. Irrespective of frequent grandstanding, quick-fix management approaches have left unresolved the most critical problems that building a highly decentralized state encompass.

12.4 References

Alvarez-Dardet C (2002). Spain. In: Marinker M, ed. *Health targets in Europe: polity, progress and promise*. London, BMJ books:76–88.

Ballart X, Ramió C (2000). *Ciencia de la Administración [Administration science]*. Valencia, Tirant Lo Blanch.

Belenes R (2003). Un balance personal de 25 años de gestión sanitaria moderna en el Sistema Nacional de Salud [A personal balance of 25 years of modern health care management in the National Health System]. *Gaceta Sanitaria*, 17(2):150–156.

Durán A, Lara JL, van Waveren M (2006). Spain: health system review. *Health Systems in Transition*, 8(4):1–208.

Ferrándiz Manjavacas FA (1999). Las Fundaciones como nuevas formas de gestión eficiente. Ventajas e inconvenientes respecto al modelo tradicional de gestión [Foundations as new modalities of efficient management: advantages and disadvantages compared with traditional management]. *Revista de Administración Sanitaria*, 3(9):33–57.

Freire JM (1998). Comentarios a propósito del documento de la Subcomisión parlamentaria para la reforma del Sistema Nacional de Salud Español [Comments in relation to the document by the Parliamentary sub-Commission on the Reform of the Spanish National Health System]. *Revista de Administración Sanitaria*, 3(9):69–92.

Freire JM (1999). Fundaciones sanitarias públicas, comentario y propuestas alternativas [Public health care foundations; comment and alternative proposals]. *Revista de Administración Sanitaria*, 2(5):23–50.

Gallego Calderón R (2002). ¿Actores o instituciones? La política sanitaria catalana [Stakeholders or institutions? The Catalan health care policy]. In Grau M, Mateos A, eds. *Análisis de políticas públicas en España: enfoques y casos [An analysis of public policies in Spain: approaches and cases]*. Valencia, Tirant lo Blanch:401–445.

García-Armesto et al. (2010). Spain: health system review. *Health Systems in Transition*, 12(4):1–287.

García-Cornejo B (2008). Información contable para la gestión en los hospitales públicos españoles: dificultades en su elaboración [Accounting information for management in Spanish public hospitals: the difficulties in getting it together]. *Gaceta Sanitaria*, 6(4):655–672.

Gómez de Hita JL (2000). *Formas jurídicas de la organización sanitaria [Legal modalities in health care organizations]*. Granada, Andalusian School of Public Health.

Guillén A, Cabiedes L (1998). La política sanitaria: análisis y perspectivas del Sistema Nacional de Salud [Health policy: analysis and perspecives of the National Health System]. In: Gomá R, Subirats J, eds. *Políticas Públicas en España. Contenidos, redes de actores y niveles de gobierno [Public poliies in Spain. Contents, stakeholders' networks and levels of government]*. Barcelona, Ariel:167–199.

Hood C (1991). A public management for all seasons. *Public Administration*, 69(1):3–19.

Marín Ferrer M, de Rosa Torner A (2007). *Las Nuevas Formas de Gestión Sanitaria "Modelo Alzira" [New health care management modalities: the "Alzira model"]*. Madrid, Instituto de Estudios Económicos.

Marín Ferrer M, de Rosa Torner A, Gómez Gómez M (2003). Modelo Alzira: concesión administrativa de servicios sanitarios públicos [The Alzira model: administrative concession of public health care services]. *Cuadernos de Gestión*, 9(4):225–233.

Martín JJ (1996). Cambios en la regulación del sistema sanitario público español: incentivos y eficiencia [Regulatory changes in the Spanish public health care system]. In: Meneu R, Ortún V, eds. *Política y Gestión Sanitaria: la Agenda Explícita [Health care management: the explicit agenda]*. Barcelona, Asociación de Economía de la Salud:177–217.

Martín JJ, López del Amo González M (2003). *Innovaciones organizativas y de gestión en el Sistema Nacional de Salud [Organizational and managerial innovations in the National Health System]*. Madrid, Spanish University for Long Distance Training.

Menéndez Rexach A (2008). La gestión indirecta de la asistencia sanitaria pública. Reflexiones en torno al debate sobre la privatización de la sanidad [Indirect management of public health care: reflections around the debate on health care privatization]. *Revista de Administración Sanitaria*, 6(2):269–296.

Sánchez Caro J (2000). Régimen Jurídico de las Nuevas Formas de Gestión en la Sanidad Pública Española (La perspectiva del Instituto Nacional de la Salud) [Legal aspects of the new management modalities in Spanish public health care (the perspective of the National Institute of Health)]. *Jornada de estudio sobre la Organización de los Servicios Públicos Sanitarios [Working sessions on public health care services organization]*. Madrid, 10–11 April, 2000.

12.5 Regulatory framework: laws, royal decree laws and royal decrees referred to in the text

Ley 7/1985, de 2 de abril, Reguladora de las bases del Régimen Local. BOE num. 80 de 03/04/1985 (http://www.boe.es/aeboe/consultas/bases_datos/doc. php?coleccion=iberlex&id=1985/05392, accessed 2 May 2011).

Ley 14/1986, de 25 de abril, General de Sanidad. BOE num. 102 de 29/04/1986 (http://www.boe.es/aeboe/consultas/bases_datos/doc.php?coleccion=iberlex& id=1986/10499, accessed 2 May 2011).

Ley 30/1992, de 26 de noviembre, de Régimen Jurídico de las Administraciones Públicas y del Procedimiento Administrativo Común. BOE num. 285 de 27/11/1992 (http://www.boe.es/aeboe/consultas/bases_datos/doc.php?colecci on=iberlex&id=1992/26318, accessed 2 May 2011).

Ley 4/1992, de 30 de diciembre, de Presupuestos de la Comunidad Autónoma de Andalucía para 1993. BOJA num. 136 de 31/12/1992 (http://www. juntadeandalucia.es/salud/sites/csalud/galerias/documentos/c_1_c_5_ normativa/normas_reguladoras_ordenacion/empresas_publicas_sanitarias/ ley_presupuestos_andalucia1993.pdf, accessed 2 May 2011).

Decreto 104/1993, de 3 de agosto, por el que se constituye la empresa pública Hospital de la Costa del Sol y se aprueban sus estatutos. BOJA num. 92 de 24/08/1993 (http://juntadeandalucia.es/boja/boletines/1993/92/d/3.html, accessed 2 May 2011).

Ley 30/1994, de 24 de noviembre, de Fundaciones y de incentivos fiscales a la participación privada en actividades de interés general. BOE num. 282 de 25/11/1994 (http://www.boe.es/aeboe/consultas/bases_datos/doc.php?colecci on=iberlex&id=1994/26004, accessed 2 May 2011).

Ley 13/1995, de 18 de Mayo, de Contratos de las Administraciones Públicas. BOE num. 119 de 19/05/1995 (http://boe.es/boe/dias/1995/05/19/pdfs/A14601-14644.pdf, accessed 2 May 2011).

Real Decreto-ley 10/1996, de 17 de junio, sobre habilitación de nuevas formas de gestión del Sistema Nacional de Salud. BOE num. 147 de 18/06/1996 (http://www.madrid.org/cs/Satellite?blobcol=urldata&blobheader=application %2Fpdf&blobheadername1=Content-Disposition&blobheadervalue1=filena me%3D44.pdf&blobkey=id&blobtable=MungoBlobs&blobwhere=1196179 678719&ssbinary=true, accessed 2 May 2011).

Ley 15/1997, de 25 de abril, sobre habilitación de nuevas formas de gestión del Sistema Nacional de Salud. BOE num. 100 de 26/04/1997 (http://www.boe. es/aeboe/consultas/bases_datos/doc.php?coleccion=iberlex&id=1997/09021, accessed 2 May 2011).

Ley 49/1998, de 30 de diciembre, de Presupuestos Generales del Estado para 1998. BOE num. 313 de 31/12/1998 (http://www.boe.es/boe/dias/1998/12/31/pdfs/A44352-44412.pdf, accessed 2 May 2011).

Ley 50/1998, de 30 de diciembre, de Medidas Fiscales, Administrativas y del Orden Social. BOE num. 313 de 31/12/1998 (http://www.boe.es/aeboe/consultas/bases_datos/doc.php?coleccion=iberlex&id=1998/30155, accessed 2 May 2011).

Real Decreto 29/2000, de 14 de enero, sobre nuevas formas de gestión del Instituto Nacional de la Salud. BOE num. 21 de 15/01/2000 (http://www.boe.es/boe/dias/2000/01/25/pdfs/A03134-03148.pdf, accessed 2 May 2011).

Ley 50/2002, de 26 de diciembre, de Fundaciones. BOE num. 310 de 27/12/2002 (http://www.boe.es/aeboe/consultas/bases_datos/doc.php?coleccion=iberlex&id=2002/25180, accessed 2 May 2011).

Ley 55/2003, de 16 de diciembre, del Estatuto Marco del Personal Sanitario de los Servicios de Salud. BOE num. 301 de 17/12/2003 (http://www.boe.es/boe/dias/2003/12/17/pdfs/A44742-44763.pdf, accessed 2 May 2011).

Ley 30/2007, de 30 de octubre, de Contratos del Sector Público. BOE num. 261 de 31/10/2007 (http://www.boe.es/aeboe/consultas/bases_datos/doc.php?coleccion=iberlex&id=2007/18874, accessed 2 May 2011).

Ley 3/2008, de 23 de diciembre, del Presupuesto de la Comunidad Autónoma de Andalucía para el año 2009. BOJA num. 259 de 31/12/2008 (http://www.juntadeandalucia.es/boja/boletines/2008/259/d/updf/d1.pdf, accessed 2 May 2011).